Springer Texts in Statisti

Springer Texts in Statistics (STS) includes advanced textbooks from 3rd- to 4th-year undergraduate courses to 1st- to 2nd-year graduate courses. Exercise sets should be included. The series editors are currently Genevera I. Allen, Richard D. De Veaux, and Rebecca Nugent. Stephen Fienberg, George Casella, and Ingram Olkin were editors of the series for many years.

More information about this series at http://www.springer.com/series/417

Ruth Etzioni • Micha Mandel • Roman Gulati

Statistics for Health Data Science

An Organic Approach

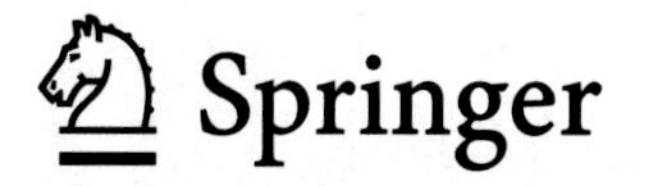

Ruth Etzioni
Fred Hutchinson Cancer Research Center
University of Washington
Seattle, WA, USA

Micha Mandel
Department of Statistics and Data Science
Hebrew University of Jerusalem
Mount Scopus, Jerusalem, Israel

Roman Gulati
Division of Public Health Sciences
Fred Hutchinson Cancer Research Center
Seattle, WA, USA

ISSN 1431-875X ISSN 2197-4136 (electronic)
Springer Texts in Statistics
ISBN 978-3-030-59888-4 ISBN 978-3-030-59889-1 (eBook)
https://doi.org/10.1007/978-3-030-59889-1

This Springer imprint is published by the registered company Springer Nature Switzerland AG
The registered company address is: Gewerbestrasse 11, 6330 Cham, Switzerland

Dedicated to the memory of Steve and Joyce Fienberg

Preface

Today's health services and health outcomes research trainees are entering a data-driven world, full of opportunities for novel research to address questions both old and new. But, this work comes with an unprecedented demand—for competence in health data science.

Health data science is multidisciplinary, encompassing statistics, health econometrics, and, now, predictive analytics. The ever-expanding universe of health data includes clinical, administrative, and population data. Each is subject to its own set of limitations, requiring researchers to be able to understand the implications for analysis and adapt accordingly. It is no wonder that cultivating competence in health data science requires covering many bases.

This text grew out of a curriculum for a core methods course offered to PhD students in health services and health outcomes at the University of Washington. Over the years, the course has also attracted students from epidemiology and global health as well as many clinician scientist trainees. Graduates of the course have told us many times that it was the most useful of their PhD classes and greatly facilitated their dissertation research. Recognizing the usefulness and uniqueness of the curriculum inspired us to create this text.

Designed for researchers who have had some exposure to the basics of statistical analysis (perhaps a first course on linear regression), this text brings together key statistical ideas that are foundational for contemporary investigators in health services, health outcomes, and health policy. We cover the classical paradigm of statistical inference, exploring regression modeling for a variety of health outcomes, where the goal is to explain. We also cross over to problems where the goal is to predict, and we discuss statistical learning and predictive analytics. We present various analyses of association appropriate for observational data, and we also study methods for causal inference. We discuss sampling and variability and how they manifest in the analysis of population surveys. In addition, we introduce bootstrapping as a tool for measuring variability in complex settings, such as the two-part model for health expenditure outcomes.

We call our pedagogical mindset *an organic approach* to convey our intent to grow understanding in a manner that feels natural. Ideally, each new concept should feel like an extension of what has come before. Our explanations are mostly non-technical and are supported by relevant stories and examples. The methods presented are applied to real-world research questions using real-world data. We explore the trends in body mass in the United States using NHANES data in Chaps. 3, 4, and 10; examine racial disparities in prostate cancer mortality using the SEER cancer registry data in Chap. 5; and quantify incremental health care costs associated with diabetes using MEPS data in Chaps. 6 and 9.

Although this text spans a wide range of ideas, models, and methods, in many ways it only scratches the surface. For each chapter, we could direct the reader to any of a number of books covering just the topic of that chapter. Moreover, there are plenty of topics that fall outside of our scope, which focuses on cross-sectional data and independent observations. Rather than being exhaustive, our goal is to provide a useful and practical foundation that students can build upon as they competently and confidently navigate the world of health data.

We thank those who encouraged and supported us in the preparation of this work. We appreciate all the students who read early chapters and encouraged us to keep writing, especially Samantha Clark and Becca Hutcheson. Noelle Noble helped with early production and with fuel toward the end. Special thanks are due to our students, Bailey Ingraham and Ernesto Ulloa-Pérez, who co-authored Chaps. 1, 2, and 4, and Marlena Bannick. We are also grateful to Daniel Nevo, Noah Simon, and David Etzioni, who read and critiqued drafts of several chapters and helped us to make them much stronger.

We thank the Department of Health Services at the University of Washington for the opportunity to teach *Advanced Research Methods* and to Steve Zeliadt and Paul Hebert, co-instructors and health services researchers from whom we learned how hard it is to define a health care cost, and who first taught us the term *recycled predictions*; to Michelle Garrison, current co-instructor and fantastic educator; and to Paula Diehr from whom one of us (RE) inherited the course and who shared the Basic Health Plan Data used in Chap. 5.

This book is dedicated to the memory of Steve and Joyce Fienberg. Steve was a giant in the field, and his vision, leadership, and impact remain constant models for us and for many statisticians. Joyce was taken from us abruptly and cruelly in the Tree of Life synagogue attack in Pittsburgh on October 27, 2018. She was the one who welcomed and embraced Steve's international students, among whom was one of us (RE). Her warmth and generosity knew no bounds.

May their memory be a blessing.

Seattle, WA, USA — Ruth Etzioni
Jerusalem, Israel — Micha Mandel
Seattle, WA, USA — Roman Gulati

Contents

List of Figures

List of Tables

Chapter 1
Statistics and Health Data

Abstract The evolution of health care data resources is creating vast new opportunities for population health research. This text is designed to guide public health students and practitioners as they navigate this changing landscape to develop competence as health data analysts. In this chapter, we define the concept of organic statistics, which will form a foundation for the methods presented in this and subsequent chapters. We differentiate between hypothesis-driven research based on classical conceptual models and predictive analytics methods that are more data-driven. We introduce the most common types of publicly available health data, and we provide examples of the types of real-world research questions that will be featured throughout the text. This chapter thus creates a roadmap for forthcoming chapters while standing alone as an introduction to the key themes of this text: health data resources and their features, the research question and its role in analysis, and the mindset of organic statistics.

1.1 Introduction

On August 4, 2014, *The Wall Street Journal* ran an article titled "In treatment, there can be too much of a good thing." The article cited two studies in which large patient databases had been used to link blood pressure and blood sugar levels with health outcomes. In the blood pressure study [1], researchers examined medical records of nearly 400,000 Kaiser Permanente patients who were taking prescription drugs for hypertension. They showed that those with lower blood pressures had higher risk of death or end-stage renal disease than those with intermediate levels. In the blood sugar study [2], researchers examined medical claims from over 33 million beneficiaries and showed that hospital admission rates for hypoglycemia had increased over time, ultimately exceeding admission rates for hyperglycemia. Attributing these trends to zealous control of diabetes, they

Coauthored by B. C. Ingraham
Department of Biostatistics, University of Washington

R. Etzioni et al., *Statistics for Health Data Science*, Springer Texts in Statistics,
https://doi.org/10.1007/978-3-030-59889-1_1

questioned whether methods for treating hyperglycemia could be improved. These two examples demonstrate the ability of statistical analyses of large databases to raise questions and to provide answers that can eventually improve our health systems.

This book is about statistics for the study of health care delivery, utilization, and outcome. We discuss different types of data resources now available to the health services researcher and explore their advantages as well as their limitations. As the universe of health data resources expands, classical statistical methods remain core, but in this book we expand our range of methods to include algorithmic approaches designed for predictive purposes and big data. We use the broad term *health care data analytics* to encompass the study of different types of contemporary data and available methods for analysis.

1.2 Statistics and Organic Statistics

There are many ways to define *statistics*. Fundamentally, statistics is how we make sense of the world through data. This happens via the process of statistical analysis. Statistical analysis translates questions into mathematical formulations or models, uses the data to learn sensible models, and, ultimately, applies the models to address the original questions. Statistics is therefore a pipeline that links question and data to answer and impact. Too often, however, statistics is identified with model fitting. This turns statistics into a collection of recipes and statistical analysis into an exercise in picking the right recipe for the data at hand. This perspective is reinforced by the wide availability of modern software packages, which permit anyone to implement any of a vast set of models at the drop of a hat.

Our vision of organic statistics is the antithesis of statistics as a collection of recipes. One of the Merriam-Webster definitions of *organic* is "having the characteristics of an organism: developing in the manner of a living plant or animal." Our objective in this text is to explain statistical methods and models so that the reader's understanding grows organically. It is not enough for researchers to know what model or method to use; they need to understand why and how it works, its advantages over other approaches in a given setting, and its underlying assumptions and limitations. While we sometimes introduce mathematical notation and expressions, our goal is to present explanations in words and pictures that make sense to a generally non-mathematical audience. We craft our explanations so that new concepts follow naturally from, and build naturally upon, what has come before. In this way, new knowledge becomes an extension of existing knowledge, culminating in a base of clear and logical understanding of statistical methods and models.

1.3 Statistical Methods and Models

This text is mostly about hypothesis-driven investigations resting on theory-based or conceptual models—an approach that is traditional in applied statistics and health services research. But we also cultivate an awareness of predictive, algorithmic approaches that are not model-based and explore some of these in the last chapter. Given the current evolution in the field of health services and health outcomes research, we feel that it is important for today's health services/health outcomes researchers to be familiar with both the traditional statistical paradigm and modern predictive ideas and methods.

In the traditional statistical paradigm, interest focuses on developing what might be called a mechanistic explanation for the observed variability in an outcome or outcomes. Here, the term *mechanistic* refers to an underlying structural phenomenon that drives heterogeneity in the data. In health care applications, the mechanism may be biological, clinical, or socio-economic. The goal is to identify it and to be able to separate it from the noise that is always present in observed data. This is the process of statistical inference, formally implemented via statistical hypothesis testing. In the traditional statistical paradigm, it is of paramount importance not to mistakenly identify mechanism when the data are being driven by random noise. We do not want to infer, for example, that a health behavior is associated with increased risk of hospitalization if individuals in the data who exhibit that behavior just happen to have more hospital stays by chance. Hypothesis testing provides a strict quantitative framework for controlling this type of error, but this framework generally rests on critical assumptions concerning the data-generating mechanism and the design of the study.

In the case of health care outcomes, traditional statistical models must account for the typically non-normal nature of the outcome variables [3]. The left-hand panel of Fig. 1.1 is a histogram of total medical expenditures for participants in the Medical

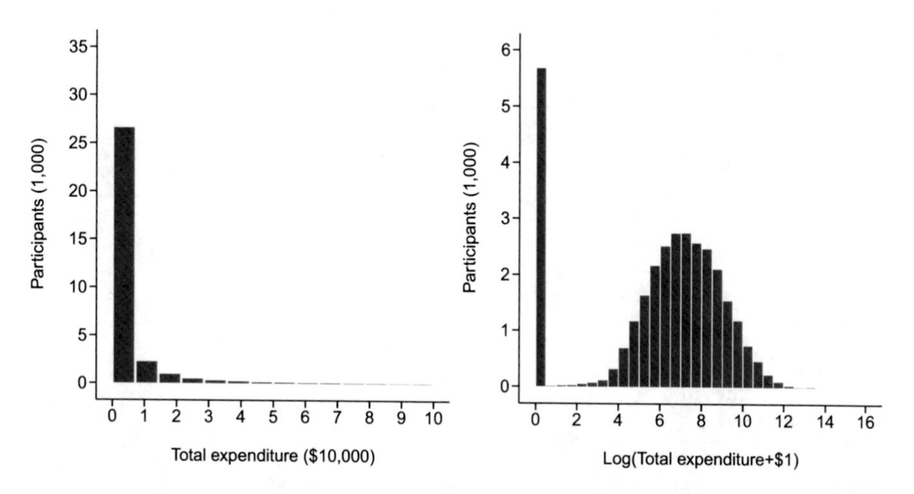

Fig. 1.1 Total annual expenditures on natural and log-transformed scales in MEPS 2017 sample data truncated at $100,000

Expenditure Panel Survey [4] in 2017. (This large health survey of households in the United States is discussed below.) Not only are the data extremely right-skewed with a long right tail but also many of the observations are zero, reflecting participants who did not record any medical care costs for that year. These two subgroups of participants are easier to see after logarithmic transformation of total expenditures, shown in the right-hand panel.

Methods appropriate for health care outcomes include linear regression, generalized linear regression models, overdispersed data models, transformation and retransformation approaches for skewed data, and two-part regression models. The majority of this book is dedicated to the study of these methods in the context of large public health databases.

Learning about mechanism is facilitated by a conceptual model that specifies the factors potentially driving the outcomes of interest and is a source for hypothesis generation. Figure 1.2 is a version of the Andersen–Newman model for health services utilization. This model partitions the drivers of utilization into predisposing, enabling, and need factors [5]. A factor's role in the conceptual model translates into a specific analytic place in the statistical model. Thus, for example, in examining hypotheses concerning the link between physical activity and health care costs, confounding factors like age or comorbid conditions should be included in the statistical model, whereas mediating factors like body mass index and self-reported

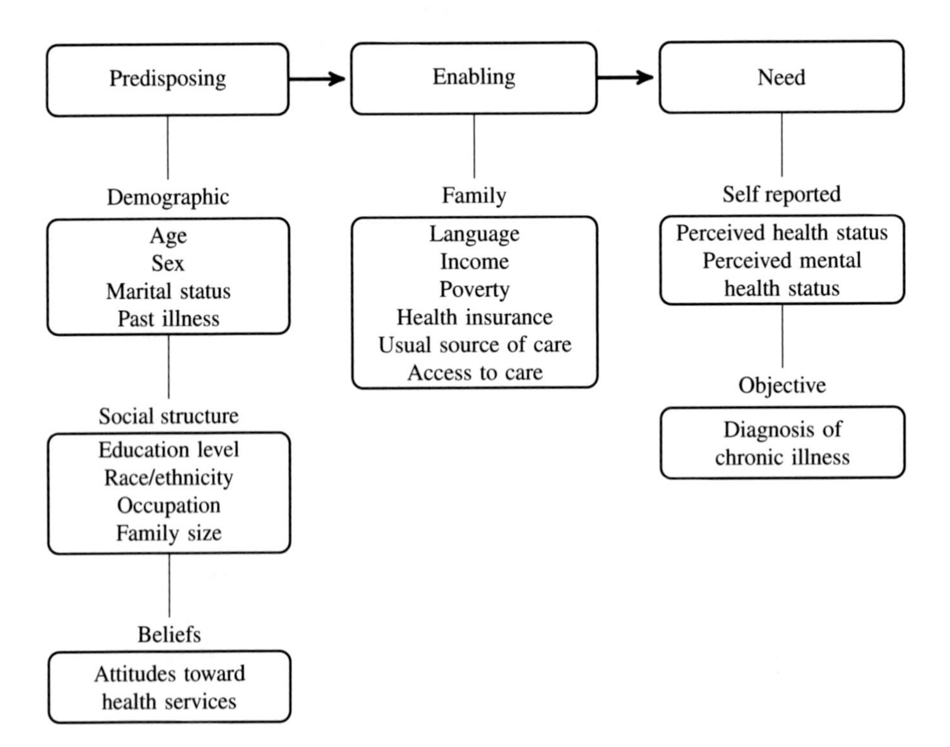

Fig. 1.2 The Andersen–Newman model for health services utilization

health may be more appropriately excluded from the statistical model. In this way, mechanism finds expression in the mathematical structure of traditional statistical models, and hypothesis testing provides a framework for making inferences about this structure, which then informs about mechanism.

The predictive analytics paradigm does not generally aim to learn about the data-generating mechanism. Rather, it learns about patterns in the data that enable predicting the outcome of interest with an accuracy that is optimal in some sense, e.g., minimizing a measure of distance between the observed and predicted outcome values. These patterns may not even be describable mathematically, and the predictive algorithm may be similarly opaque.

Algorithmic methods are relatively novel in the health services and outcomes literature; but, given their usefulness and their growing importance in health research, we introduce them and compare them with traditional statistical approaches in key examples. The predictive analytics paradigm is much less structured and generally makes fewer assumptions than traditional statistical approaches, but it does not lend itself to inference about specific factors that might be impacting individuals' health, and therefore it may not provide direction for specific interventions to improve outcomes.

To make these ideas concrete, consider the example of predicting hospitalizations. This was the objective of the Heritage Provider Network (HPN) prize [6], one of the first examples of crowdsourcing biomedical data analytics solutions. Since the original HPN prize competition, there have been dozens of biomedical analytics competitions and challenges.

The HPN prize aimed to develop an algorithm for predicting how many days a patient would spend in a hospital in a year given three prior contiguous years of claims and demographic data. The competition started in April 2011 and offered over $3 million in prizes. It attracted more than 16,000 data scientists, who submitted more than 25,000 models; these were evaluated at regular intervals ("milestones") to provide comparative performance metrics (based on mean squared error in a target dataset) for the entries.

What kinds of models made it to the top? For the first three milestones, papers describing the approaches used by the top entrants are provided on the HPN prize website [7]. The "Market Makers" paper after the first milestone [8] cites four different predictive modeling algorithms, and final predictions were based on an *ensemble* or combination of the predictions from each one. Thus, although the final model performed well in that it minimized a distance criterion between the observed and predicted outcomes, it was not actually interpretable in terms of associations between any of the predictors and the outcome. The algorithm was able to tell you who was most likely to be hospitalized in the coming year, but it could not tell you why. How to intervene clinically to prevent the adverse outcome was therefore not immediately apparent despite the model's predictive superiority.

Which approach is to be preferred—the one that aims to identify mechanism or the one that aims to predict outcome? The answer depends on the objective of the analysis and how the results are to be used in practice. In some cases, the choice is clear cut; in others, it is not. When a scientific question is hypothesis-driven and investigates a specific mechanism or cause potentially driving the outcome in a target population, the analyst may be naturally drawn to a traditional statistical approach. However, even in such a setting, the predictive accuracy of the model may be of interest, particularly when the choice of regression model is not obvious a priori. We comment on valid inference post model selection when we review the perils of making inferences after stepwise regression (Chap. 10).

In this text, we cover mostly traditional approaches, but we also explore algorithmic predictive approaches as we address a variety of real-data research questions. Our objective is to expose the reader to a broad range of analytical questions and different analytical mindsets in the hope that this will foster a well-founded personal philosophy of health data analytics.

1.4 Health Care Data

In this section, we review the types of health care data available for research into the drivers of health care utilization and outcomes. We first distinguish between *administrative* and *non-administrative* data. Administrative data are collected as a matter of course for the financial and administrative aspects of health care delivery. These data include medical claims and electronic medical records. They are valuable because they have the potential to provide an objective snapshot of the care delivered. However, these data are generally not collected for research purposes [9], and many challenges arise when using them to address research questions. Some organizations assemble administrative data for research purposes; an example is the Health Care Utilization Project [10], which samples and curates encounter-level health care data in the US and packages these data for researchers. Non-administrative data sources include registries and surveys. These data are gathered for surveillance or research purposes, yet they too have many limitations stemming from the manner in which they are collected.

Each data type provides an opportunity to address a range of research questions. As a health data analyst, it is important to match a given research question to the data resource that is most likely to provide a valid answer. Table 1.1 is our attempt to summarize information that is typically provided with each data type. Different data types may be linked to provide a more comprehensive record.

Some questions can be addressed using multiple data types. Consider, for example, the problem of estimating the prevalence of hypertension in a specified population. This information could be extracted from population surveys that specifically ask participants whether they have been previously diagnosed with the condition. Or it could be identified from medical claims that bill for encounters or medications is associated with a hypertension diagnosis code. Alternatively, it could be obtained from electronic medical records, which provide measurements of patients' health status including (frequently) blood pressure.

Each of these sources is subject to its own caveats and limitations. In a comparison [11] of the prevalence of hypertension assessed via different sources—

Table 1.1 Data categories typically available in each type of health care data source. Dots indicate low (gray) and high (black) reliability with respect to comprehensiveness of data at the individual level

Data category	Medical claims	Medical records	Surveys	Registries
Socio-demographics	•		•	•
Medical histories	•	•	•	•
Hospitalizations	•	•	•	
Outpatient care	•	•	•	
Medical expenditures	•		•	
Health behaviors			•	
Diagnoses	•	•	•	•
Procedures	•	•		•
Medications	•	•	•	•
Diagnostic test results		•	•	•

surveys, medication records, and blood pressure measurements, none provided a complete picture. Estimates based on these distinct data sources each yielded a population prevalence of approximately 30%, but a substantial fraction of cases assessed via each of these indications did not overlap with cases assessed by the other indications. It is important to understand which individuals are represented in each data source and adjust or interpret the analysis in light of over-, non-, or under-represented groups. And it is critical to understand the data-generating process in each setting. Below we briefly summarize some key characteristics—and implications—of the data-generating process for medical claims, medical records, health surveys, and disease registries.

1.4.1 Medical Claims

Medical claims code the billable interactions between insured patients and the health care delivery system. The purpose of a claim is to generate payment from the payer for the services provided. Thus, a medical claim includes the information needed to justify the claim and quantify its expense.

A *claim* is a structured form that lists diagnosis and procedure codes, prescribed medications, and medical care costs. For diagnoses, most facilities in the US use the International Classification of Diseases (ICD) coding system. This coding system is revised periodically; in 2015, the system underwent a major transition from ICD-9 to ICD-10, which expanded the number of unique diagnosis codes almost fivefold to over 68,000 codes. *Procedure codes* describe the services rendered to patients. There are several coding systems for procedures. The ICD-10 system includes codes for inpatient procedures. The Current Procedure Terminology (CPT) codes and the Healthcare Common Procedure Coding System (HCPCS), which builds on the CPT codes, describe procedures conducted as part of outpatient or ambulatory care. Many CPT and HCPCS codes overlap, but HCPCS codes also capture non-physician services, such as ambulance rides, durable medical equipment use, and prescription drug use.

How is a medical claim produced? In practice, trained claims coders extract the relevant information from the medical record and clinical documentation. Then, this information is translated into insurance claims and bills for patients. Given the complexity of the diagnosis and procedure coding systems, it can be challenging to properly code an encounter. On top of the resulting uncertainty, the same service may be billed differently depending on the payer. A *New York Times* article [12] cited an example of two friends who got drive-through coronavirus tests at the same emergency center in Austin and received very different bills depending on whether they paid cash ($199) or billed their test to their health insurance company ($6408).

Although medical claims are generated for billing purposes and not for research, they contain a wealth of information that pertains to important research questions about delivery of care, disparities in care, and the effectiveness and quality of care. Hence, claims databases are increasingly being used for research purposes. These databases are generally payer-specific, although commercial products that aggregate claims from multiple payers are becoming more available. Since claims are generated for billing, they should be analyzed with an awareness of the kinds of incentives that exist in this setting, which may skew the recording of care received in claims data.

Claims data have many limitations. Only insured patients can be studied using claims databases, and only covered services are represented. Thus, claims data are not broadly population representative, and they are by nature incomplete; for example, information on non-prescription drugs is lacking. Further, claims can only be recorded if patients are enrolled in a health care plan and are missing if coverage lapses or if they switch to a different payer. Claims data must therefore be studied in the context of health plan enrollment, which may change over time.

While claims data are frequently used to analyze health care utilization, key predictors such as socio-demographic and socio-economic factors are generally not available at the individual level; this may limit predictive and causal studies. Claims data are also frequently used to learn about patterns of care for a specific condition, but because of the wide variability in how claims are coded, such analyses invariably underascertain individuals with that condition. In general, the sensitivity and specificity of medical claims can be limited, particularly when the target population is somewhat nuanced, e.g., identifying cancer cases with a specific disease stage or distinguishing Type I and Type II diabetes.

A major limitation of medical claims is that they do not include health status measurements or diagnostic test results. The blood sugar study mentioned above [2] focused on hospital admissions for hyper- and hypoglycemia; by identifying these conditions on the basis of the discharge diagnosis, it could be conducted using medical claims. However, if a measurement of blood sugar level had been required to confirm the diagnosis, the study would have needed access to the patients' medical records. We discuss medical records as a data resource in the next section.

It can be difficult to get access to medical claims data without a formal proposal, funds, and (in some cases) a demonstrably effective data security protocol. To allow researchers to gain familiarity with their data structures, the Centers for Medicare and Medicaid Services offers synthetic public use files (SynPUFs) on Medicare claims for download [13]. Ability to access private payer claims is very limited without direct collaboration with a payer or an integrated health system. Some private payers are packaging their claims as commercial data products and licensing them to research institutions for a fee. However, the procedures for licensing the data, the specific agreements and costs involved, and the data representation and quality can differ considerably across available products.

1.4.2 Medical Records

Medical records contain comprehensive electronic clinical data obtained at the point of care. They are used to track health conditions, interventions, and outcomes at the individual patient level for the purpose of diagnosis and treatment.

Medical records include the same structured diagnosis and procedure information as in medical claims. However, medical records include all patients who received care regardless of insurance status and incorporate much richer information on the health status of the patients and their care. This includes unstructured data, such as physician notes, imaging reports, vital status measurements, and diagnostic test results. The Kaiser Permanente blood pressure study [1] identified patients based on whether they had a diagnosed condition and were on prescribed medication for this condition; in addition, the study required measurement of achieved blood pressures. Thus, this work could only be done using medical records.

Medical records offer tremendous potential for understanding processes of care, researching effectiveness of interventions, and predicting health outcomes in real-world settings. In addition, the possibility of real-time prediction based on data analytics of medical records has generated enormous excitement, with implications for creating real-time alerts and identifying novel strata of patient risk. However, like claims, medical records are not generated for research purposes, and their limitations must be understood.

The first limitation concerns data quality. Weiskopf and Weng [14] formulate five metrics to help researchers assess medical record quality: completeness, correctness, concordance (with other sources), plausibility, and currency (or timeliness). The second limitation relates to the problem of phenotyping—identifying a diagnosis, procedure, or outcome from a medical record. Because the record is formed from multiple data streams, including structured and unstructured fields, the seemingly simple act of identifying populations or events may in practice require an algorithm to learn from the available data elements and reconcile them. If the algorithm is not highly sensitive and specific, the resulting misclassification can lead to biases in estimated associations and predictions.

From an analytic perspective, a medical record is a real-time surveillance instrument that does not follow a statistical design or plan. Whether information is recorded or not may be linked with the underlying condition of the patient. Sicker patients generally have more diagnostic tests or more frequent vital status assessments than healthier patients. These realities may lead to informative missing data patterns, which may bias estimates of associations between predictors and outcomes.

While the potential for medical record data to advance health research is clear, raw medical record data are generally proprietary to their health system and are not routinely accessible to outside researchers. These data include highly sensitive information about individuals who are protected by the Health Insurance Portability and Accountability Act; therefore, the majority of medical record data are available for research only on a limited, tightly controlled basis. However, data from medical records are exported and curated to many other agencies. There are public resources, like the Comprehensive Hospital Abstract Reporting System [15], National Inpatient Sample [16], Substance Abuse and Mental Health Services Administration facility data [17], and commercial data collections, that can be accessed with a research proposal and fees.

1.4.3 Health Surveys

Health surveys record patients responses to sets of questions designed to learn about a wide range of correlates of population health. These include socio-demographics, health behaviors and conditions, and access to care and utilization patterns. Here, we review three large national publicly available health surveys.

The National Health Interview Survey (NHIS) [18] is the nation's largest in-person household health survey. Since 1957, the NHIS has been conducted annually by the Census Bureau on behalf of the National Center for Health Statistics (NCHS). The survey is cross sectional and collects information on a different sample every year. The NHIS questions cover a wide variety of topics, including medical conditions, health insurance, doctor visits, and health behaviors. Results from the NHIS have been used to monitor trends in the burden of chronic conditions and health care access and to track progress toward national health objectives.

The National Health and Nutrition Examination Survey (NHANES) [19], also conducted by the NCHS, goes one step further than the NHIS in that it not only interviews participants but also includes a full physical examination and blood test. While this step is logistically complex and adds significant cost, it yields objective measurements of important health indicators, such as blood pressure, body mass index, and hemoglobin A1c. NHANES data have been crucial in providing the data to create growth charts for children, monitor the prevalence of obesity and overweight, and estimate the frequency of undiagnosed diabetes in the US. National policies to eliminate lead in gasoline and food resources grew out of NHANES results. Similarly, ongoing national programs to reduce hypertension and cholesterol levels depend on NHANES data to target education and prevention efforts.

The Medical Expenditure Panel Survey (MEPS) [4] conducted by the Agency for Healthcare Research and Quality collects extensive information on health care utilization and expenditures for a subsample of NHIS households. In addition to key socio-demographic, health history, and health behavior variables from NHIS, MEPS also includes detailed health insurance information as well as data on inpatient, outpatient, and prescription drug utilization, along with the corresponding expenditures sourced from medical providers and health records. MEPS is a rolling panel survey that enrolls participants annually and interviews them five times over a period of 2 years. Thus, in contrast to NHIS and NHANES, which are cross sectional, MEPS provides longitudinal information for a limited duration on each participant. MEPS data have been useful in tracking health care expenditures, identifying the most costly medical conditions, and monitoring the use of and costs of different types of care in the population.

All of the aforementioned surveys are designed with complex sampling and weighting schemes to reduce the costs of survey administration and produce results that are population representative. Rather than performing simple random sampling, survey designs include stratification to control the proportion sampled within population subgroups and clustering to control survey costs. Each observation in a survey is associated with a weight that reflects the number of individuals in the target population represented by that observation. Survey documentation provides sampling scheme and weight estimation details and can be important in informing data analyses. It is important to understand these details and to track any changes in survey design over time, which may, in turn, generate changes in analytic results. The sampling scheme is taken into account by incorporating the survey design and weights into the analysis. Software packages like R and Stata include commands and survey analysis packages for this purpose.

Many of the examples in this book use MEPS data. These data provide a rich environment for exploring topical health services questions while demonstrating specialized methods and techniques relevant for observational health care databases. Although MEPS follows a complex survey design, these aspects are ignored until we present analytic methods that account for survey design variables (Chap. 9).

Surveys are of enormous value because they directly query respondents for information that may be difficult or impossible to obtain from administrative data, such as socio-demographic characteristics, health behaviors, and individual perceptions and preferences. At the same time, surveys are subject to a host of potential biases stemming from the very nature of survey research and the way it queries and interacts with the population [20]. Potential biases include non-response bias, recall bias, and social desirability bias. All of these can skew survey responses and/or lead to non-representative survey samples. Mitigation of these biases requires extensive development and calibration of survey instruments and careful consideration of the mode of survey implementation.

1.4.4 Disease Registries

A registry is a corpus of non-administrative data collected for population surveillance of a specific condition or group of conditions. In the US, there are registries for cancer, end-stage renal disease, Alzheimer's disease, and Down syndrome, to name a few. Registries have a clearly specified objective, a set of variables designed to address the objective, and an infrastructure to collect the desired data items. Unlike population surveys, registries are generally not random samples; some, like the Alzheimer's Prevention Registry [21], are opt-in datasets; others, like the Surveillance, Epidemiology, and End Results (SEER) registry [22] of the National Cancer Institute, are a complete census in certain regions.

The SEER registry is an example of an established population disease registry. SEER collects information on all diagnosed cancer cases within a specific set of catchment areas (subregistries) in the US. The objective of the SEER registry is to track the burden of cancer incidence and mortality in the population. Once new cases have been identified, a set of patient- and disease-specific factors is abstracted by hospital-based cancer registrars. These factors include individual-level demographics, some socio-economic data at the census-tract level, disease characteristics, and first course of cancer-directed therapy. Following diagnosis, information about survival and cause of death is obtained via linkage to vital status records from the NCHS.

The SEER registry is an indispensable tool for researchers and others interested in understanding how the profile of cancer is changing over time. SEER data have registered dramatic changes in prostate cancer incidence following the advent of the prostate-specific antigen test for prostate cancer, declines in cervical cancer incidence after the introduction of pap smears, and a persistent, still not completely understood climb in the incidence of melanoma. SEER results are also critical in setting priorities for cancer prevention and control programs and for assessing the nation's success in attaining healthy population goals as they relate to cancer [23].

Data quality and representativeness are two potential limitations of disease registry data. Opt-in registries, such as the Alzheimer's Prevention Registry [21], are naturally subject to selection factors, which will affect representation. The SEER registry is a complete census within defined catchment areas in the US, so its representativeness is determined by the catchment population.

With any data source, it is important to investigate whether there are specific processes to assure data quality, reliability, and completeness. In SEER [24], reliability studies measure consistency in the application of coding rules across registry sites by providing multiple coders with a reference set of medical records and assessing agreement of their results. Case-finding audits ensure that all eligible cases are being identified and that cancer incidence rates are accurate. These are just some examples of work that can be done to ensure quality of registry data.

As a population surveillance instrument, a registry will be affected by changes in how disease cases are defined and ascertained. If diagnostic modalities used to define and detect disease become more accessible or more sensitive with time, then incidence may appear to be on the rise solely due to increased detection of disease. In some cases, definitions of disease may change; in 2017, the American College of Cardiology and American Heart Association changed the criteria for classifying patients as hypertensive to include a systolic blood pressure of 130 mm Hg or more, replacing the previous threshold of 140 mm Hg, and leading to an expectation that the prevalence of high blood pressure would triple among men under age 45 and double among women under age 45 [25].

To the extent that registries are created in service to specific objectives, the scope of the data that they collect may be limited. The focus of the SEER registry on cancer incidence has led to a data infrastructure that is based on pathology reports and includes information that pertains to disease diagnosis. This may be acceptable for cancer incidence, but it is not adequate for cancer recurrence, which is often identified by medical imaging. A linkage between SEER registry records and medical claims is available for Medicare beneficiaries via the linked SEER-Medicare database [26]. This linked data resource has informed a host of investigations relating to treatment patterns and post-diagnosis outcomes among cancer patients in the US.

1.5 Outline of the Text

The rest of this text is organized as follows. In Chap. 2, we begin with basic statistical background and hypothesis testing that will prove useful in later chapters. In Chap. 3, we review standard linear regression modeling with special emphasis on ways to include variables with different roles in a conceptual model. We also introduce quantile and non-parametric regression.

Since many health care outcomes are binary or categorical in nature, Chap. 4 presents a suite of methods for analyzing such data and introduces the *recycled prediction* [27] approach for marginal effect estimation, which we will use repeatedly to transform results of non-linear models to the scale of the response variable. Chapter 5 covers count data outcomes and includes discussion of overdispersed and zero-inflated methods. Chapter 6 moves on to the analysis of skewed cost data, including two-part models. These methods do not make the usual assumptions of ordinary least squares; they accommodate skewed cost data that may include a spike at zero.

Chapter 7 introduces the ideas of resampling and bootstrapping and uses these techniques to summarize uncertainty in two-part models. This is followed in Chap. 8 by a discussion of causality, causal inference, and strengths and limitations of different designs for observational studies of health care outcomes. Chapter 9 presents a detailed discussion of designs used for health surveys and how to account for the design in the analysis of survey data. Finally, Chap. 10 takes a second look at some of the applied examples studied in previous chapters using a predictive modeling perspective and introduces some statistical learning algorithms potentially useful in health services and outcomes research. In all chapters, methods are illustrated via topical examples of research questions in the health services and health outcomes literature.

There are many books about statistical models and health econometrics methods and a growing number of books about data science. In this book, we bring together key ideas and techniques from all of these disciplines and apply them to the questions of health services and outcomes today. By using real data from large publicly available resources, we demystify the process of dealing with health data and provide a practical roadmap for contemporary health data analytics.

1.6 Software and Data

R code to download data and to carry out the examples in this book is available at the GitHub page, https://roman-gulati.github.io/statistics-for-health-data-science/. Our example analyses relied heavily not only on the R language and base packages [28] but also on several R packages designed to facilitate reading, manipulating, visualizing, summarizing, and modeling data [29–37].

References

1. Sim, J.J., Shi, J., Kovesdy, C.P., Kalantar-Zadeh, K., Jacobsen, S.J.: Impact of achieved blood pressures on mortality risk and end-stage renal disease among a large, diverse hypertension population. J. Am. Coll. Cardiol. **64**, 588–597 (2014)
2. Lipska, K.J., Ross, J.S., Wang, Y., Inzucchi, S.E., Minges, K., Karter, A.J., Huang, E.S., Desai, M.M., Gill, T.M., Krumholz, H.M.: National trends in US hospital admissions for hyperglycemia and hypoglycemia among Medicare beneficiaries, 1999 to 2011. JAMA Intern. Med. **174**, 1116–1124 (2014)
3. Diehr, P., Yanez, D., Ash, A., Hornbrook, M., Lin, D.Y.: Methods for analyzing health care utilization and costs. Annu. Rev. Public Health **20**, 125–144 (1999)
4. Agency for Healthcare Research and Quality: Medical Expenditure Panel Survey. http://www.ahrq.gov/research/data/meps/index.html. Accessed 12 Feb 2020
5. Andersen, R., Newman, J.F.: Societal and individual determinants of medical care utilization in the United States. Milbank Mem. Fund Q. Health Soc. **51**, 95–124 (1973)
6. Heritage Provider Network: National Heritage Prize. http://www.heritagehealthprize.com/c/hhp. Accessed 12 Feb 2020
7. Heritage Provider Network: National Heritage Prize Milestone Winners. http://www.heritagehealthprize.com/c/hhp/details/milestone-winners. Accessed 12 Feb 2020
8. Brierley, P., Vogel, D., Axelrod, R.: Heritage Provider Network health prize round 1 milestone prize: how we did it—team "market makers" (2013). https://foreverdata.org/1015/content/milestone1-2.pdf. Accessed 12 Feb 2020
9. Casey, J.A., Schwartz, B.S., Stewart, W.F., Adler, N.E.: Using electronic health records for population health research: a review of methods and applications. Annu. Rev. Public Health **37**, 61–81 (2016)
10. Agency for Healthcare Research and Quality: Healthcare Cost and Utilization Project. https://www.hcup-us.ahrq.gov/. Accessed 12 Feb 2020

11. Peng, M., Chen, G., Kaplan, G.G., Lix, L.M., Drummond, N., Lucyk, K., Garies, S., Lowerison, M., Weibe, S., Quan, H.: Methods of defining hypertension in electronic medical records: validation against national survey data. J. Public Health **38**, e392–e399 (2016)
12. Kliff, S.: Two friends in Texas were tested for coronavirus. One bill was $199. The other? $6,408 (2020). https://www.nytimes.com/2020/06/29/upshot/coronavirus-tests-unpredictable-prices.html. Accessed 11 July 2020
13. Centers for Medicare & Medicaid Services: Medicare Claims Synthetic Public Use Files. https://www.cms.gov/Research-Statistics-Data-and-Systems/Downloadable-Public-Use-Files/SynPUFs. Accessed 12 Feb 2020
14. Weiskopf, N.G., Weng, C.: Methods and dimensions of electronic health record data quality assessment: Enabling reuse for clinical research. J. Am. Med. Inform. Assoc. **20**, 144–151 (2013)
15. Washington State Department of Health: Comprehensive Hospital Abstract Reporting System. https://www.doh.wa.gov/ForPublicHealthandHealthcareProviders/HealthcareProfessionsandFacilities/DataReportingandRetrieval/HospitalInpatientDatabaseCHARS. Accessed 12 Feb 2020
16. Agency for Healthcare Research and Quality: National Inpatient Sample. https://www.hcup-us.ahrq.gov/nisoverview.jsp. Accessed 12 Feb 2020
17. U.S. Department of Health & Human Services: Substance Abuse and Mental Health Services Administration. https://www.samhsa.gov/. Accessed 12 Feb 2020
18. Centers for Disease Control and Prevention: National Health Interview Survey. http://www.cdc.gov/nchs/nhis/index.htm. Accessed 12 Feb 2020
19. Centers for Disease Control and Prevention: National Health and Nutrition Examination Survey. https://www.cdc.gov/nchs/nhanes/index.htm. Accessed 12 Feb 2020
20. Lavrakas, P.J. (ed.): Encyclopedia of Survey Research Methods (2008). https://doi.org/10.4135/9781412963947
21. Banner Alzheimer's Institute: Alzheimer's Prevention Registry. www.endalznow.org. Accessed 19 July 2020
22. National Cancer Institute: Surveillance, Epidemiology, and End Results. http://seer.cancer.gov/registries/. Accessed 12 Feb 2020
23. U.S. Department of Health & Human Services: Healthy People 2020. https://www.healthypeople.gov/2020/topics-objectives/topic/cancer. Accessed 12 Feb 2020
24. National Cancer Institute: SEER Quality Improvement. https://seer.cancer.gov/qi. Accessed 12 Feb 2020
25. American College of Cardiology: New ACC/AHA High Blood Pressure Guidelines Lower Definition of Hypertension. https://www.acc.org/latest-in-cardiology/articles/2017/11/08/11/47/mon-5pm-bp-guideline-aha-2017. Accessed July 30 2020
26. National Cancer Institute: SEER-Medicare Linked Database. http://healthcaredelivery.cancer.gov/seermedicare/. Accessed 12 Feb 2020
27. Kleinman, L.C., Norton, E.: What's the risk? A simple approach for estimating adjusted risk measures from nonlinear models including logistic regression. Health Serv. Res. **44**, 288–302 (2009)
28. R Core Team: R: A Language and Environment for Statistical Computing. R Foundation for Statistical Computing, Vienna, (2020). https://www.R-project.org/
29. Wickham, H., Francois, R., Henry, L., Müller, K.: dplyr: A Grammar of Data Manipulation (2020). https://CRAN.R-project.org/package=dplyr. R package version 0.8.5
30. Wickham, H., Hester, J., Francois, R.: readr: Read Rectangular Text Data (2018). https://CRAN.R-project.org/package=readr. R package version 1.3.1
31. Wickham, H.: tidyverse: Easily Install and Load the 'tidyverse' (2017). https://CRAN.R-project.org/package=tidyverse. R package version 1.2.1
32. R Core Team: foreign: Read data stored by 'Minitab', 'S', 'SAS', 'SPSS', 'Stata', 'Systat', 'Weka', 'dBase', ... (2020). https://CRAN.R-project.org/package=foreign. R package version 0.8-76

33. Wickham, H.: ggplot2: Elegant Graphics for Data Analysis. Springer, New York (2016). https://ggplot2.tidyverse.org
34. Wickham, H., Seidel, D.: Scales: Scale Functions for Visualization (2019). https://CRAN.R-project.org/package=scales. R package version 1.1.0
35. Garnier, S.: viridis: Default Color Maps from 'matplotlib' (2018). https://CRAN.R-project.org/package=viridis. R package version 0.5.1
36. Dahl, D.B., Scott, D., Roosen, C., Magnusson, A., Swinton, J.: xtable: Export Tables to LaTeX or HTML (2019). https://CRAN.R-project.org/package=xtable. R package version 1.8-4
37. Müller, K.: here: A Simpler Way to Find Your Files (2017). https://CRAN.R-project.org/package=here. R package version 0.1

Chapter 2
Key Statistical Concepts

Abstract This chapter offers a statistics boot camp for the study of data on health care outcomes. These outcomes are frequently not normally distributed and require specialized modeling and regression techniques. After reviewing basic statistical concepts, we introduce statistical distributions commonly used to model health outcomes. We explain conditional and marginal estimation, discuss between-individual heterogeneity, and recommend strategies for working with heavy-tailed distributions. We conclude with a review of hypothesis testing and a discussion about inference in small—and big—data settings.

2.1 Samples and Populations

Statistics is the way we make inferences from a sample about a defined population. We begin our discussion by defining these fundamental concepts.

Population The main goal of health research is to learn about health outcomes and their drivers in the population. This is the aim of clinical trials and most observational health care studies. We should therefore be very clear about the population to which research findings apply. The population can be well defined at the outset, e.g., all people who were in the city of Hiroshima at the time of the atomic bombings and survived the first year, or can be hypothetical, e.g., all breast cancer patients who have undergone or will undergo radical mastectomy. The researcher must be able to determine if a subject belongs to the defined population.

A sub-population is a population in and of itself that satisfies well-defined properties. In the above examples, we may be interested in the sub-population of men under the age of 20 years or patients with hormone-receptor-positive breast cancer who have undergone radical mastectomy. Many scientific questions relate to differences between sub-populations; for example, comparing treated and untreated

---

Coauthored by E. Ulloa-Pérez
Department of Biostatistics, University of Washington

R. Etzioni et al., *Statistics for Health Data Science*, Springer Texts in Statistics,
https://doi.org/10.1007/978-3-030-59889-1_2

groups to determine whether treatment is beneficial. Regression models, introduced in detail in Chap. 3, concern sub-populations as they estimate the mean outcome for different groups (sub-populations) defined by the covariates.

Sample A sample is a subset of the population that is used to learn about that population. In contrast to a sub-population that is defined by fixed criteria, a sample is generally selected via a random mechanism. Random sampling enables the scientist to make inference about the population and, importantly, to quantify uncertainty around the results. Survey samples are examples of random samples, but many observational studies are not randomly sampled. They may be samples of convenience, such as single-institution cohorts, which consist of all patients treated for a specific condition at that institution. Or they may be a complete census, such as cancer registries, which include all cancer cases diagnosed in their catchment area. Regardless of how samples are obtained, their use to learn about a target population means that issues of representativeness are inevitable and deserve to be addressed.

2.2 Statistics Basics

2.2.1 Random Variables

The study of health care outcomes is the study of the random variables that measure these outcomes. A random variable captures a specific characteristic of individuals in the population, and its values typically vary across individuals. Each random variable can take on a range of values in theory although, in practice, we observe a specific value for each individual. Examples of random variables that are health outcomes include the following:

- Whether a patient is hospitalized or re-admitted after surgery
- Whether a breast cancer patient receives a mastectomy or a lumpectomy
- Types of prescription medications filled for a specific condition
- Days hospitalized after a specific type of surgery
- Inpatient, outpatient, or prescription medication expenditures within a year
- Number and types of advanced imaging tests after primary cancer treatment
- Number of outpatient visits over a defined time interval
- Total annual expenditures among patients within a specific health category.

When referring to random variables generically or theoretically, we use capital letters like X and Y. When referring to specific values, we use small letters like x and y. Thus, for example, we might talk about an unspecified patient age X with a range from 20 to 85 years, but for a given patient, we might observe a specific age x equal to 62 years.

2.2.2 Dependent and Independent Variables

A key first task in any analysis is to identify the dependent (Y) and independent (X) variables. Dependent variables are also called *outcome* or *response* variables, and independent variables are also called *predictors* or *covariates*.

In regression analyses, the central question concerns how Y changes as X varies. More precisely, if the value of the independent variable X changes, then what is the consequence for the dependent variable Y? Loosely speaking, the independent and dependent variables are analogous to "cause" and "effect," where the quotation marks here emphasize that this is just an analogy, and that cause must be rigorously determined using an appropriate study design and analysis.

Whether a variable is an independent or a dependent variable depends on the research question. It can sometimes be quite challenging to decide which variable is dependent and which is independent, particularly when there are feedback loops going in both directions between the variables. For instance, suppose you are investigating the association between elective vigorous exercise and insomnia. Research has suggested that exercise (done at the right time of the day) may reduce insomnia. But insomnia may also reduce a person's ability to exercise.

Sometimes, outcomes other than the one specified may masquerade as potential independent variables. For example, suppose you are studying how medical expenditures in a given year depend on smoking history. Based on the scientific question, the independent variable is smoking history and the dependent variable is medical expenditures. But suppose we also have information on the number of hospitalizations in the same year. The number of hospitalizations will be strongly correlated with medical expenditures, but for this question both hospitalizations and medical expenditures are best considered as dependent variables that coevolve. A carefully considered conceptual model like the Andersen–Newman model [1] that was introduced in Chap. 1 can be very useful to sort out the independent and dependent variables in an analysis.

2.2.3 Statistical Distributions and Their Summaries

Each random variable has a distribution that describes the probability that the variable takes any value in its range.

A categorical variable can take any of a finite number of discrete values, and the distribution is given by a finite set of probabilities corresponding to these possible values, with the probabilities summing to 1.

A continuous variable has many (effectively an infinite number of) possible values. Consequently, the probability of each value is very small. In principle, we can imagine the distribution of a continuous variable as an extremely detailed histogram in which the widths of the intervals become very small. The histogram becomes a curve called the *probability density function* (PDF) of the random variable, and the area under the PDF over any interval represents the probability that the random variable will have a value within that interval. The *cumulative distribution function* (CDF) at a specified value gives the probability that the random variable takes on a value smaller than or equal to that value and is mathematically equal to the integral of the PDF up to that value.

Words used to describe the shape of a distribution include *symmetric*, *skewed*, *heavy-tailed* or *kurtotic* (referring to a high frequency of extreme values), and *uni-* or *multimodal* (referring to the number of peaks of the most likely values).

Quantitative summaries of distributions often focus on identifying the most typical, or representative, value of a random variable. The *mean* (also called *average* or *expected value*) is perhaps the most commonly cited measure of a typical value. The mean of a random variable Y is denoted by $E(Y)$. Other common summaries are *percentiles* or *quantiles*, which describe values according to where they lie within the CDF. The *median* is the 50th percentile and represents the center of the distribution in the sense that 50% of the observations are below it and 50% are above it. The median and the mean coincide if the distribution is symmetric and differ otherwise; the mean is influenced by extreme (large and small) observations, while the median is not. Health care outcomes are often right-skewed because of the presence of a few heavy users whose health is extremely poor relative to the rest of the population. In such cases, the mean is larger than the median, and therefore the median may be a better summary of a typical value of the population.

Figure 2.1 is a histogram of total costs among persons with any reported inpatient costs based on data from the Medical Expenditure Panel Survey (MEPS) in 2017 [2]. The MEPS collects information on socio-demographics, health behavior, health insurance, health care utilization, and expenditures for a population-representative sample of households in the United States. Although MEPS involves a complex

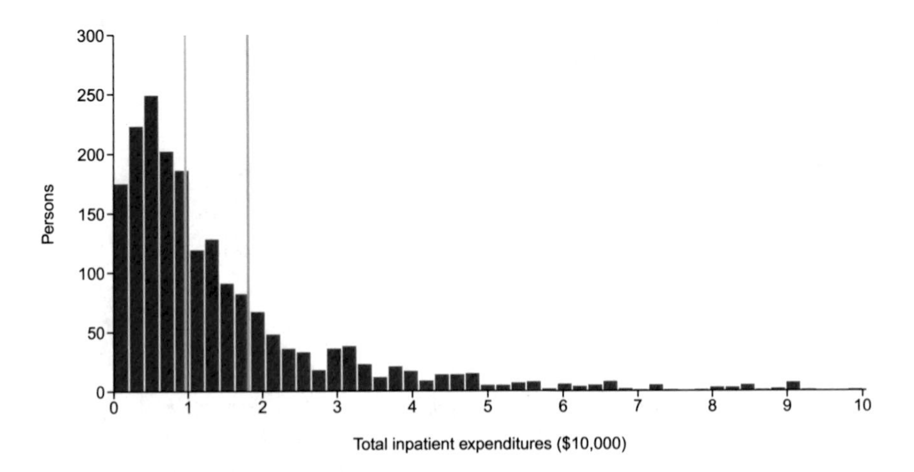

Fig. 2.1 Histogram of total inpatient expenditures among persons with any inpatient expenditures in the MEPS 2017 sample data truncated at $100,000. Vertical lines show mean (orange) and median (blue)

survey design, including stratified, clustered random sampling and survey weights, in this chapter we restrict attention to the sample participants and postpone discussion of these topics to Chap. 9. The figure shows an extreme right-skewed distribution with a mean of $18,145 and a much lower median of $9664.

2.2.4 Parameters and Models

Without further specification, a distribution may refer to a whole family of distributions. Parameters, typically denoted by Greek letters like μ and α, allow us to specify which member of the family we are talking about. Thus, we can talk about a random variable having a normal distribution, but by specifying the mean $\mu = 9.8$ and the variance $\sigma^2 = 2.4$, we narrow focus to a specific normal distribution.

Parametric statistical methods specify the family of distributions and then use the data to learn about its specific member by estimating the parameters. If f is the PDF of an outcome variable Y, interest may focus on its mean and variance. In regression analysis, we try to explain how the parameters of f depend on covariates X. In classical linear regression, we assume that Y has a normal distribution with mean $\mu = E(Y)$, and we estimate how $E(Y)$ depends on X. Because many health care outcomes do not follow a normal distribution, we introduce distributions that are more appropriate for these outcomes later in this chapter. Non-parametric methods do not specify a family for f. Non-parametric methods for regression are discussed in Chap. 3, and a specific non-parametric test for comparing population summaries, a permutation test, is presented in Chap. 7.

The term *model* is ubiquitous in statistics. The model comprises the assumptions and mathematical specifications for the analysis. The model depends on the data and the research question, but it is rarely unique; in most cases, there is more than one model that might reasonably address the same question given the data. In predicting annual medical expenditures based on the MEPS, for example, the model specification includes the set of candidate covariates, the mathematical expression linking the predictor variables with the expenditure outcome, and any assumptions about the distribution of the outcome. The question of what constitutes a good model is one that we will return to repeatedly in this book.

2.2.5 Estimation and Inference

Estimation is the process by which the sample is used to learn about the population. The sample mean is a natural estimate of the population mean, and the sample median is a natural estimate of the population median. When we talk about estimating a population summary measure (sometimes referred to as a *population parameter*) or estimating the distribution of a random variable, we are talking about using the data to learn about these features in the population.

Statistical inference is the process by which sample estimates are used to answer research questions and address specified hypotheses about the population. Thus, for example, the *sample mean* is an estimate, the *sample standard error* is an estimate, and a hypothesis test is a procedure by which these estimates are combined to make inferences. We discuss hypothesis tests as tools for statistical inference in the last section of this chapter.

2.2.6 Variation and Standard Error

Estimates are functions of the sampled data. Although we always observe only a single sample, we must take into consideration the fact that it was randomly drawn among many potential samples. Thus, we can think about an estimate as having a distribution that reflects its variation over repeated samples.

The standard error of an estimate quantifies the variation that we would expect if we could repeat the sampling and modeling that generated the estimate many times. Technically, the standard error is measured by the standard deviation of the estimate. The standard deviation ($\text{SD}(Y)$) of a variable Y is the square root of the *variance*, which measures the average (squared) distance between the values of Y and its mean. While the SD is used as the natural measure of variability, having the same physical units as Y, the variance is more convenient for mathematical calculations.

The standard error of an estimate is a function of the sample data, the formulation of the estimate, and the variability of the observations. A higher standard error implies that we would expect greater variation if we could repeat the sampling and estimation many times. A sample of 10 randomly selected Y values from a population will produce a higher standard error around an estimate than a sample of 100 randomly selected Y values.

The standard error of an estimate is also a function of the model used. Different models may yield similar estimates but produce different standard errors. In later chapters, we will discover that standard linear models produce similar regression estimates of incremental medical expenditures as more complex *two-part models* (Chap. 6) but with potentially very different standard errors. Since the standard error is an important component of any hypothesis test based on the estimate, the specific model used can impact inferences made.

Confidence intervals place estimates in the context of their standard errors; they are sometimes referred to as *interval estimates*. Like standard errors, confidence intervals are interpreted in terms of what we would expect if we could repeat the sampling and estimation many times. In the case of a 95% confidence interval for the mean, the appropriate interpretation is: if the sampling and estimation could be repeated many times, an interval so constructed would include the true mean 95% of the time. Interpretation of confidence intervals can be challenging because a specific interval is estimated but it is interpreted in terms of the underlying sampling and estimation process.

2.2.7 *Conditional and Marginal Means*

In health care studies, we are frequently interested in comparisons of outcomes (Y) in sub-populations defined by values of random variables (X). The *conditional mean* of Y given $X = x$, denoted $E(Y \mid X = x)$, is the mean for the sub-population with the specific value (x) of the predictor variable (X).

Table 2.1 shows estimated total medical expenditures per person (Y) for MEPS 2017 participants according to perceived health status at the start of the year (X), ranging from "Excellent" to "Poor." The table also provides the percentage of respondents falling into each health category corresponding to the size of each sub-population.

According to Table 2.1, the conditional mean expenditures given "Excellent" health are $E(Y \mid X = \text{"Excellent"}) = \$1957$ and the conditional mean expenditures given "Poor" health are $E(Y \mid X = \text{"Poor"}) = \$22{,}619$. As might be anticipated, medical expenditures are strongly dependent on perceived health status; worse health is associated with higher expenditures. If a person had "Excellent" health, one would predict very different annual expenditures than if that person had "Poor" health.

What if we wanted to predict a person's total medical expenditures without knowing his or her perceived health status? What would be the most reasonable way to form a prediction? In this case, assuming that the person in question was representative of the population, their likelihood of belonging in each health category would be given by the corresponding percentage in the table. So a reasonable guess for their expenses would be the *weighted average* of the conditional means, with weights given by those percentages. This average of the conditional means is called the *marginal mean* $E(Y)$ because it no longer conditions on X; rather, it averages over the distribution of X. In Table 2.1, the marginal mean, calculated by the weighted average, is:

$$E(Y) = 1957 \times 0.34 + 3729 \times 0.29 + 6183 \times 0.25 + 11387 \times 0.10 + 22619 \times 0.03.$$

This is equal to \$5110. This might seem low when compared with the highest expenditures in the table, but this is because persons with better health, who have correspondingly lower expenditures, were more frequent in the sample than persons in poorer health. This concept of a marginal mean extends also to other

Table 2.1 Total medical expenditures per person in MEPS 2017 by perceived health status

Perceived health status	Percentage of sample	Total expenditures
Excellent	34%	$1957
Very good	29%	$3729
Good	25%	$6183
Fair	10%	$11,387
Poor	3%	$22,619

statistics, such as the variance, and even to distributions. Thus, we may talk about the *conditional distribution* of Y given $X = x$ if we want to study the sub-population defined by $X = x$, and, by extension, the marginal distribution of Y if we are interested in the whole population.

2.2.8 *Joint and Mixture Distributions*

Joint distributions come about when two or more random variables vary together, e.g., when two outcome variables coevolve in a dependent fashion. An example of this phenomenon might be total medical care costs and hospitalizations over a specified interval. In cases where we have multiple coevolving outcomes, we do not generally try to estimate the conditional mean of one outcome given another. Rather, we model them together as a multivariate outcome.

Mixture distributions arise when one part of the data follows one distribution and the other part follows another distribution. Two-part models can be used to study a type of mixture distribution for medical expenditures where one part of the sample (a fraction p) has no medical expenditures because they have not accessed the health care system and the other part of the sample (a fraction $1 - p$) has expenditures that follow a specified distribution.

Figure 2.1 is a histogram of total costs among persons with any reported inpatient costs based on MEPS 2017 data. The figure shows an extremely right-skewed distribution that also has a high frequency of low values; this distribution can be modeled as a two-part mixture distribution with a spike at zero reflecting the fraction of the sample incurring zero health care expenditures for the year (see Chap. 6).

2.2.9 *Variable Transformations*

Transformation of a random variable can play a useful role in a statistical analysis. Consider a random variable Y with PDF f, and suppose we have a general function of Y, $G(Y)$. Some functions that will be of interest, particularly in studying health care expenditures, include the *logarithmic* transformation ($G(Y) = \log(Y)$) and the *exponential* transformation ($G(Y) = \exp(Y)$). How does applying G change the distribution of Y and its summaries such as the mean, variance, and percentiles? The answer, in general, is that it depends on G.

If G is a linear function, i.e., $G(Y) = aY + b$, then there are known formulas for the mean and variance of $G(Y)$; namely, $E[G(Y)] = aE(Y) + b$ and $\text{Var}[G(Y)] = a^2\text{Var}(Y)$. If G is a non-linear function, then it can completely change the distribution of Y and alter its mean and variance in ways that require customized study.

We discuss the case of the non-linear logarithmic and exponential transformations later in this chapter and in Chap. 6. When G is one of these transformations, the following are true:

1. If M is the median of Y, then $G(M)$ is the median of $G(Y)$, and similarly for other percentiles.
2. If p is the probability that Y falls in an interval (a, b), then p is also the probability that $G(Y)$ falls in the interval $(G(a), G(b))$.

Thus both percentiles and probability are translated by these transformations. In fact, (1) and (2) are true for any increasing transformation.

2.3 Common Statistical Distributions and Concepts

In this section, we introduce several key statistical distributions and concepts that serve as useful foundations for the development of parametric regression models introduced in subsequent chapters.

2.3.1 *The Bernoulli and Binomial Distributions for Binary Outcomes*

The first example of health care outcomes given earlier in this chapter was binary in nature: whether a patient is re-admitted after surgery. The Bernoulli distribution is the family of distributions for a binary outcome Y that can take on values 0 and 1. We will refer to these as negative and positive outcomes, respectively, reflecting non-occurrence or occurrence of an event of interest.

Binary regression analysis focuses on $P(Y = 1)$, the probability that Y will take the value 1, and attempts to identify factors X that are associated with that probability. In our example, this means studying the factors that are associated with higher versus lower risks of re-admission. When the Bernoulli distribution is used, it turns out that $P(Y = 1)$ is in fact the mean of Y; thus, the problem of learning about the correlates X of $P(Y = 1)$ is essentially the same as the problem of modeling the conditional mean $E(Y \mid X)$.

Predicting a binary outcome is a version of a *classification* problem in which observations fall into two classes and the objective is to identify the combination of factors X that best predicts class membership. This perspective on the binary prediction problem is prevalent in the statistical learning literature, which has its own collection of algorithms for classification problems. We discuss the differences between this approach and the traditional statistical approach in Chap. 10.

Some important features of the Bernoulli distribution include the following:

- Even though there are two outcomes in the binary setting, the frequency distribution of the outcome is completely determined by the probability of one of the outcomes, conventionally taken to be $p = P(Y = 1)$, because the probability of the alternative outcome is $1 - p$. Classical statistical inference is concerned with identifying predictors X associated with the likelihood of Y taking the value 1 rather than 0. The odds of Y being 1 (rather than zero) are written as $p/(1-p)$. Logistic regression, discussed in Chap. 4, identifies predictors of higher versus lower odds of Y taking the value 1.
- The mean of Y, $E(Y)$, is p. Since the range of Y is from zero to one, the mean is somewhere in between.
- The variance of Y, Var(Y), is $p(1 - p)$. Thus, the variance is not independent of the mean as is the case with the normal distribution. Instead, there is a very specific relationship between the mean and the variance.
- When we have a set of n independent Bernoulli variables, the total number of positive outcomes has a binomial distribution, and this total has mean np and variance $np(1-p)$. Thus, the total number of re-admissions after surgery at a specific hospital might be binomial, where n is the number of surgeries performed at that hospital. Figure 2.2 shows several binomial distributions with different n and p.
- The binomial distribution only results from a set of Bernoulli variables if the total number n is fixed, and only if the Bernoulli variables are independent. If we are considering the number of re-admissions given the total number of surgeries performed at a specific hospital, the requirement of independence may be violated by the clustering of patients within surgeons; in this case, patients treated by the same surgeon may be more similar to one another in terms of their risk of re-admission than patients treated by other surgeons. This kind of clustering induces correlation between patients treated by the same surgeon.

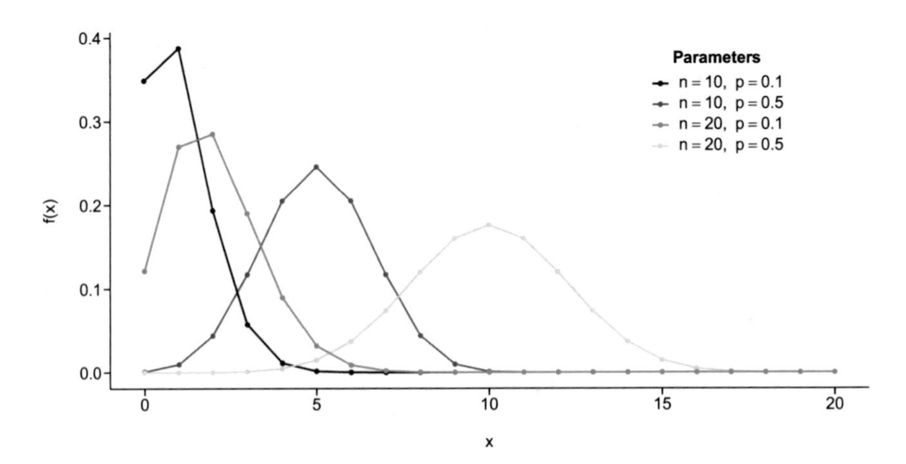

Fig. 2.2 Binomial probability function for different values of n and p. The binomial random variable can take on only non-negative integer values smaller than or equal to n; the lines in the figure are plotted for ease of presentation; actual probabilities are shown as dots

2.3.2 *The Multinomial Distribution for Categorical Outcomes*

The multinomial distribution is a generalization of the binomial to the setting where there are multiple types of outcomes beyond just positive or negative. One example might be the case of treatment choice when there are more than two treatments, such as surgery, radiation, or hormonal therapy for cancer. Another might be the case of responses to a survey question about health status, with responses being on a five-point scale. In the first example, we would describe the outcome as multinomial with three (unordered) categories. In the second example, we could describe the outcome as multinomial with five (ordered) categories.

As in the binomial setting, attention focuses on the probabilities or frequencies of each category or, equivalently, the probability that Y falls into each category. In the binary setting, we considered p and $1 - p$; in the multinomial setting, we have multiple ps—as many as the possible values of Y. However, the probabilities must add up to 1 because each observation must fall into one of the categories. Thus, in the case of K categories, the distribution has $K - 1$ parameters. The multinomial distribution of self-reported health status on a five-point scale would have four independent categories.

Multinomial regression is concerned with identifying the factors that predict the likelihood of an outcome being in one category rather than another. Thus, for example, in studying how a diabetes diagnosis impacts self-reported health, we would want to understand how $P(Y = k)$, the probability that Y will take on category k, changes depending on diabetes status.

2.3.3 *The Poisson and Negative Binomial Distributions for Counts*

In the study of health care outcomes, we often study counts: numbers of doctor visits, numbers of prescriptions filled, or numbers of procedures of a specific type performed in a facility over a month or a year.

The most basic parametric distribution for count data is the Poisson distribution. The Poisson distribution describes the probability that a count of events in a given time interval will be zero, one, two, and so on. It is derived theoretically by considering a setting in which events occur at a constant rate in a memoryless fashion (i.e., the chance that an event will occur within a specified interval is independent of the time elapsed since the last event). The Poisson distribution is the distribution of the number of such events in a specified time interval. Figure 2.3 graphs several Poisson distributions with different means.

One important feature of the Poisson distribution is that its mean and variance are equal. This, together with the basic assumptions upon which it is based, makes the Poisson distribution highly restrictive for modeling count health data. In practice, counts of medical events and procedures almost never satisfy the assumptions that

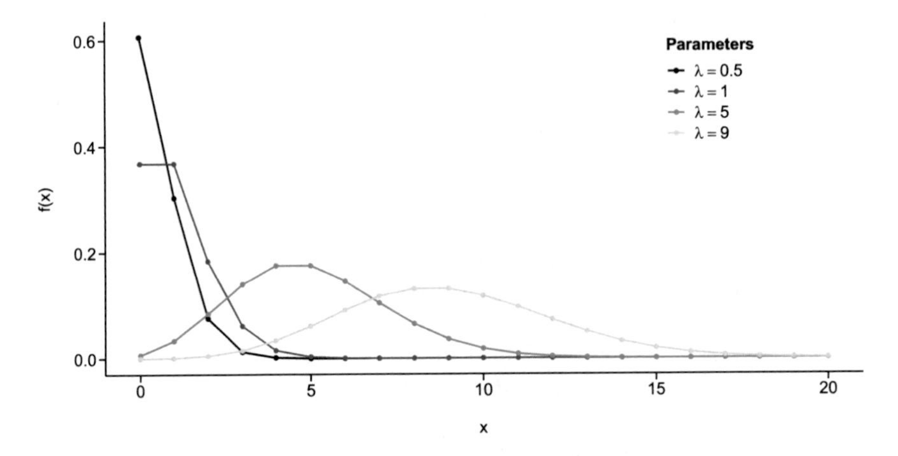

Fig. 2.3 Poisson probability function for different values of the mean λ. The Poisson random variable can take on only non-negative integer values; the lines in the figure are plotted for ease of presentation; actual probabilities are shown as dots

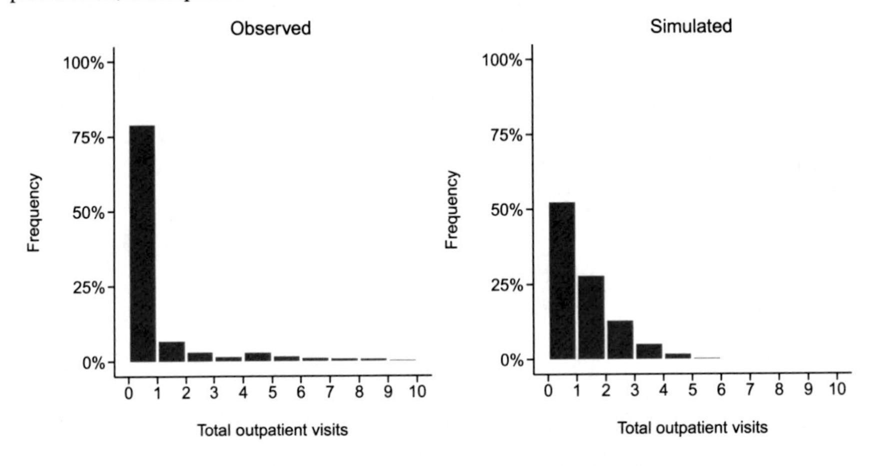

Fig. 2.4 Histograms of observed outpatient visits among participants with previous diagnosis of a stroke in the MEPS 2017 sample data (left) and simulated outpatient visits using a Poisson distribution with the same mean number of visits as the observed data. Both histograms are truncated at 10 visits

generate a Poisson distribution. Most often, the variance of a count outcome is considerably larger than its mean value.

Figure 2.4 is a histogram of outpatient visits among participants who reported a previous diagnosis of a stroke in the MEPS 2017 data. The histogram for the observed data is graphed next to a histogram reflecting a Poisson distribution with the same average number of visits (1.5). The observed data histogram shows higher frequencies at the extremes of the range, with considerably more patients with no visits and a longer right tail than the Poisson data histogram. In fact, the variance of the observed number of visits is 24, more than 15 times greater than the observed mean. We say that the observed number of visits is *overdispersed*.

When a count outcome is overdispersed, we look to an alternative model for count data that accommodate a variance that is larger than the mean. The negative binomial distribution provides such an alternative. Like the Poisson, it is appropriate for discrete, non-negative outcomes, but, unlike the Poisson, its variance always exceeds its mean.

The mechanism of overdispersion that leads to the negative binomial distribution arises from considering that individuals are heterogeneous in their count data outcomes in a manner that goes beyond observed predictors. When modeling outpatient visits, for example, one could imagine that each individual has a latent susceptibility that relates to the frequency with which they seek care in the outpatient setting. Those individuals with low susceptibility would be expected to seek care rarely and have few or no outpatient visits, and those with high susceptibility would have many visits.

Formally, we can think of each person having a Poisson-distributed count outcome Y, but, rather than everyone having the same mean μ, each individual, indexed by i, has their own mean, which may be written as μr_i. Here, i indexes individuals and r_i is a latent, individual-specific multiplier, sometimes called a *frailty*, that modifies the overall mean and personalizes it. We say that a person's conditional mean given r_i is μr_i, and since the count outcome for person i is Poisson distributed, the conditional variance for person i is also μr_i. These are conditional means and variances since they are subject-specific and differ among individuals in the population. They incorporate the notion of individual heterogeneity and add variability to the marginal distribution of Y. The negative binomial arises as the marginal distribution of Y under a very specific distribution for the r_i. It turns out that if the r_is have a gamma distribution (described below) with mean 1 and variance α, then the marginal distribution of Y is negative binomial with mean μ and variance $\mu(1 + \alpha\mu)$.

Mathematically, this result shows that latent heterogeneity in a Poisson setting will generate overdispersion and, under specific assumptions about the form of the heterogeneity, will produce a negative binomial rather than a Poisson distribution.

In practice, the negative binomial is often preferred over the Poisson for modeling count data outcomes due to its greater flexibility and ability to accommodate overdispersion. It should be remembered that the negative binomial model for count data is also quite specific in that it captures a particular mechanism—between-individual heterogeneity—for the overdispersion and makes specific assumptions about how this heterogeneity manifests in the population.

The notion that between-individual heterogeneity might lead to inflation of overall variance arises over and over again in the analysis of health outcomes. The representation of this heterogeneity via a latent, individual-specific factor that varies across individuals according to a specified distribution is the foundation for random effects and frailty models in the settings of clustered, longitudinal, and failure-time outcomes. Mathematical details aside, the way in which this additional heterogeneity affects overall variability is the same across settings. Allowing individuals to deviate from a common mean outcome in a personalized way changes the spread of the marginal distribution of the outcome. The histogram of the outcome expands to reflect a greater frequency of more extreme outcomes (from individuals with very low and very high frailties) and leads to greater mass in the tails of the distribution as illustrated in the left panel of Fig. 2.4. This is what we mean by overdispersion relative to the Poisson distribution.

2.3.4 The Normal Distribution for Continuous Outcomes

This distribution is symmetric and defined by two parameters: the mean, which is the center of symmetry, and the standard deviation, which is a measure of the variability of the values around the mean. Figure 2.5 shows several normal distributions with mean $\mu = 0$ and different values for the SD σ. About 67% of the observations occur within one SD and about 95% occur within 2 SDs of the mean. In many contexts, being more than 2 SDs from the mean is considered an atypical observation, and being 3 or more SDs from the mean is considered an "outlier."

If Y has a normal distribution with mean μ and standard deviation σ, we call $Y - \mu$ the *centered* variable and $Z = (Y - \mu)/\sigma$ a *standardized* variable. The standardized variable has mean 0 and SD 1; in fact, this is true even if the distribution is not normal. If Y is normal, we call the distribution of Z the standard normal distribution. The percentiles of Z are regularly used for statistical inference and can be found in published tables or by using appropriate functions in statistical software.

Henri Poincaré is reputed to have said that mathematicians believe in the normal distribution because it is a fact of observation, and observers believe in it because it is a theorem of mathematics. While the normal model approximates the distribution of many random variables, such as height or weight, it is by no means the optimal model for most health care outcomes. However, it is one of the most important

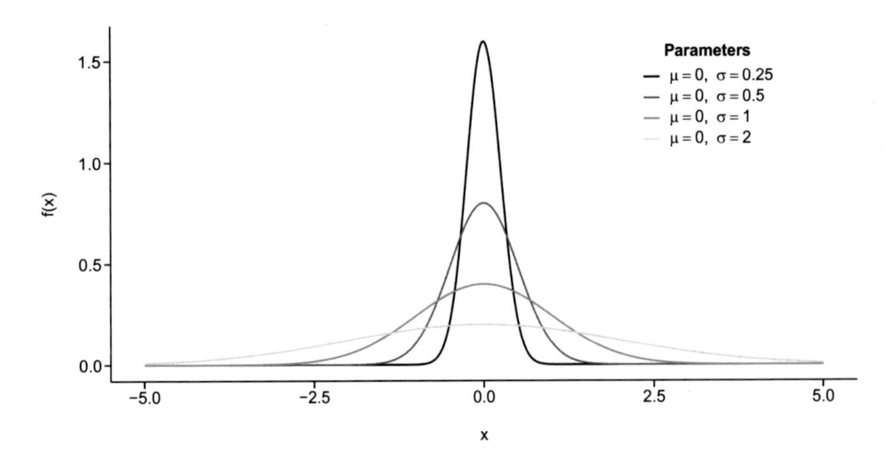

Fig. 2.5 Normal density for different values of σ

distributions to know because of the *central limit theorem*. This theorem implies that the distribution of sums of large numbers of independent random variables can be approximated by a normal distribution. Practically, this implies that the distribution of the sample mean and many of the parameter estimates that we will encounter are well approximated by the normal distribution. This important property is leveraged in many hypothesis tests used for inference. Note that this property pertains to the sample estimates and not to the population data distribution. This is perhaps one of the most remarkable and useful facts in statistics—while the values obtained in the sample can have any distribution, their average can generally be assumed to have a normal distribution.

2.3.5 *The Gamma and Lognormal Distributions for Right-Skewed Outcomes*

The gamma distribution is a distribution that is appropriate for non-negative, continuous outcomes and can capture distributions that are highly right-skewed, like medical expenditures. Figure 2.6 graphs different gamma distributions and demonstrates the flexibility of the functional form. The functional form is defined by two parameters, which we will denote by α and β. The mean of the gamma distribution is α/β and the variance is α/β^2. Thus, the variance is related to the mean and can be greater than or less than the mean, depending on the value of β.

A second distribution commonly used for modeling right-skewed outcomes is the lognormal. A variable has a lognormal distribution if its log has a normal distribution. Framed another way, the lognormal distribution arises from exponentiating a normal random variable. If Y has a $N(\mu, \sigma^2)$ distribution, then we say that $\exp(Y)$ has a lognormal distribution with parameters μ and σ^2. Its mean is not $\exp(\mu)$ but rather:

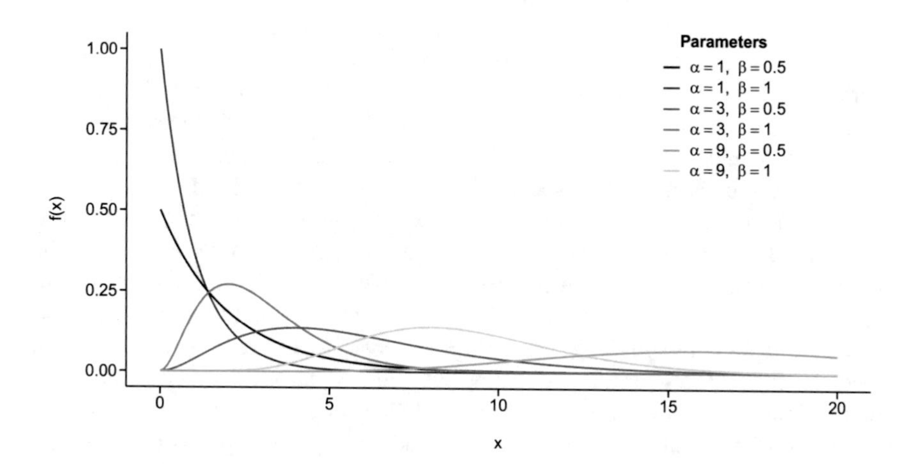

Fig. 2.6 Gamma density for different values of α and β

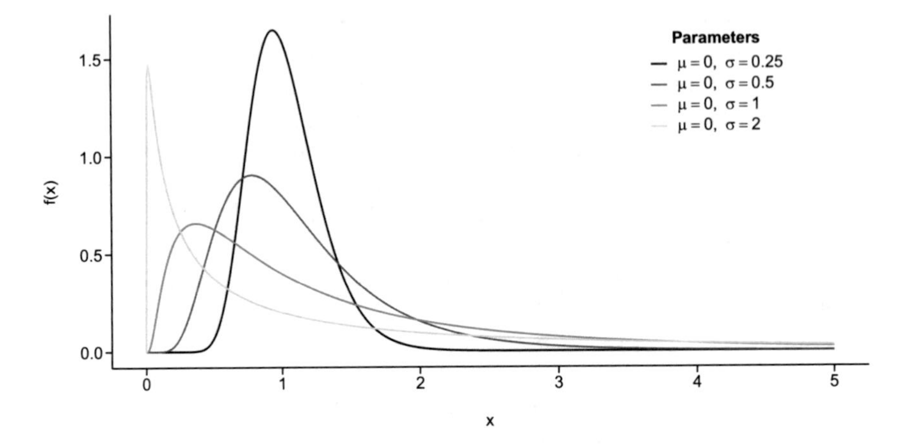

Fig. 2.7 Lognormal density for different values of σ

$$E\left[\exp\left(Y\right)\right] = \exp\left(\mu + \frac{1}{2}\sigma^2\right).$$

Figure 2.7 graphs several lognormal distributions. The figure shows the PDFs for $\exp(Y)$, where the mean of Y is zero and the standard deviation of Y varies from 0.25 to 2.

Any regression analysis that logs the dependent variable before running the regression is implicitly assuming the outcome follows a lognormal distribution. This is because logging the outcome variable and then conducting a regression analysis based on the normal distribution equates to assuming that the original outcome (before logging) is lognormal.

The lognormal distribution was traditionally favored for modeling medical costs because it can have a heavy-tailed distribution, well suited for capturing a non-trivial frequency of exceptionally large observations. But a persistent problem encountered by analysts using this model is that their regression estimates and inferences all pertain to "log dollars" and that retransforming regression coefficients to the metric of dollars is not always straightforward. We will revisit this problem later in the context of regression analysis for medical care costs, but here we illustrate the retransformation issues with respect to the mean using the MEPS data.

Suppose Y reflects the log of a health expenditure outcome, and the mean of Y is μ. What is the mean of expenditures? One might be tempted to suggest that the mean must be $\exp(\mu)$. But this would not be correct. Table 2.2 demonstrates this using medical costs from the MEPS 2017 data. The table has three columns of mean estimates corresponding to three types of costs: total, inpatient, and outpatient medical expenditures for the year. Some subjects had zero expenditures for one or more of these outcomes, and they were excluded for simplicity. The first column corresponds to the observed costs. The second column corresponds to the logged costs. And the third column simply exponentiates the second column. In our

Table 2.2 Total, outpatient, and inpatient medical expenses per person in MEPS 2017 calculated directly, after log-transformation, and after retransformation

Expense type	Total expenses	Logged expenses	Retransformed expenses
Total	$5995	7.27	$1433
Outpatient	$2767	6.59	$728
Inpatient	$18,145	9.10	$8967

notation, the first column represents $E(Y)$, the second column $E[\log(Y)]$, and the third column $\exp\{E[\log(Y)]\}$.

Although mathematically $E(Y) = \exp\{\log[E(Y)]\}$, the third column does not get us back to the first column. We cannot simply exchange the calculation of the mean of a variable and its log; the order of the operations is important. Indeed, in each case, the first column is greater than the third column, reflecting the general relationship:

$$E(Y) = E\{\exp[\log(Y)]\} \geq \exp\{E[\log(Y)]\}.$$

In fact, when we exponentiate a normal random variable, the mean depends not only on the mean of the original random variable but also on its variance. Formally, if $E[\log(Y)] = \mu$ and $\mathrm{Var}[\log(Y)] = \sigma^2$, then:

$$E(Y) = \exp\left(\mu + \frac{1}{2}\sigma^2\right) = \exp(\mu) \times \exp\left(\frac{1}{2}\sigma^2\right).$$

We discuss the implications of the retransformation issue for data analysis of medical expenditures in Chap. 6. If the log-transformed outcome is truly normally distributed, the median is not affected by the order of operations, and the median of $\exp(Y)$ is equal to $\exp[\mathrm{median}(Y)]$. Thus, an alternative to modeling the mean of Y in this setting would be to use a quantile regression model discussed in Chap. 3.

2.4 Hypothesis Testing and Statistical Inference

Hypothesis testing is the most well-known—and the most controversial—tool for statistical inference. We have defined inference as the process by which sample estimates are used to answer research questions and address specified hypotheses about the population.

Hypothesis testing is a statistical procedure that is used to reach a yes–no decision about a hypothesis based on a sample estimate of the quantity of interest (e.g., the sample mean or a regression coefficient). In practice, however, things are not so clear cut. The uncertainty in the sample means that decisions cannot be made unequivocally; there is always a chance that the decision made will turn out not to be correct. Therefore, a more accurate definition of hypothesis testing is that it is a statistical procedure used to reach a decision about a hypothesis based on a sample *while quantifying the risk that the decision made is wrong*.

In practice, a hypothesis test is a one-way street, permitting only one decision: rejection of a specified (null) hypothesis H_0, which is typically set up to be the opposite of what we wish to investigate. For example, if we hypothesize that inpatient expenditures depend on self-reported health, we would set up our null hypothesis H_0 to be that these two random variables are not associated. Rejecting H_0 would amount to "proving" our hypothesis. We reject H_0 if the sample data appear to contradict it; specifically, if our estimate is not close to the hypothesized value. The core of the hypothesis testing procedure is to control the chance that this is a mistake.

To calculate the chance of mistakenly rejecting H_0, we assume that the null hypothesis is indeed correct. Then, we calculate the p-value, which is the probability of obtaining an estimate as *or more extreme* than that observed, where more extreme means further away from H_0. A low p-value means that our estimate is not consistent with H_0. In this case, we infer that there is only a small chance that the data we observed were generated under the null hypothesis and therefore a correspondingly low chance of being wrong by rejecting it. If the p-value is small enough (e.g., less than 0.05), we reject the null hypothesis and cite the p-value as a measure of the strength of evidence in support of this decision.

Users of hypothesis testing are often prone to over-interpretation of the p-value, citing it as the likelihood that H_0 is true [3, 4], when all it can capture is the extent to which the observed data are inconsistent with H_0. Note the difference between these two interpretations: the first is a statement about the hypothesis, and the second is a statement about the data. Classical hypothesis testing does not permit direct statements about H_0 and the likelihood it is true. We can only make statements about the data and their likelihood under H_0. In fact, the one-way structure of the procedure only permits inferring that the observed data are *inconsistent* with H_0. There is no converse; we cannot infer that the observed data are consistent with H_0, even if the p-value is large. In this case, we can only issue a statement that we do not have evidence to reject H_0. In hypothesis testing, absence of evidence is not the same as evidence of absence. Needless to say, this can be rather unsatisfying.

Many of the issues with hypothesis testing arise from the wide adoption of a standard for a "small enough" p-value that has led to misinterpretation and even manipulation of the results of such tests. The historical convention is that a p-value below 0.05 is "statistically significant" and justifies rejection of the null hypothesis. However, comparing a p-value against a universal standard is highly problematic, and many professional societies and organizations have disavowed this practice in recent years [e.g., 5].

What are the problems with a standard 0.05 threshold for a p-value? For one thing, p-values may be small even in the absence of practically significant evidence against the null hypothesis. This frequently occurs when sample sizes are very large, as is the case in many publicly available health care databases. It is not uncommon in such settings to obtain an estimate of the coefficient of interest that is close to zero but has a tiny p-value. Conversely, p-values may be larger than 0.05 even when the observed evidence against the hypothesis is compelling. This happens most often when the sample is small and there is enough uncertainty that we cannot tell whether the observed data are really inconsistent with H_0. We say that the *power* of the test is inadequate, where power is defined as the probability of correctly rejecting H_0 if it is indeed false. Power is closely linked to sample size, and an important step in planning or designing a study is to make sure that the sample size is large enough so that practically important departures from H_0 can be detected.

The existence of a standard 0.05 threshold can lead to manipulation when there are incentives to rejecting H_0. A dataset can be "p-hacked" by applying multiple methods or models and then reporting only the results of those that lead to a small p-value without reporting the others. Methodological manipulations may involve choosing convenient exclusion criteria (e.g., restricting to subjects within a certain age range), choosing a specific metric for variables (e.g., dichotomizing a continuous covariate at a carefully selected cut point), choosing how to process data (e.g., dropping subjects with certain kinds of missing data), or using a specific test (e.g., performing a t-test rather than a non-parametric Wilcoxon test). By making certain choices, p-values can be manipulated to produce results that end up being statistically significant. It is reasonable to apply multiple methods to confirm robustness of any inferences, but these should all be reported, particularly if they do not all produce the same conclusion.

A further issue is that the information provided by a p-value depends on the number of tests conducted [6]. When there are multiple comparisons made in a dataset, the chance of at least one producing a small p-value increases. Analyses involving multiple comparisons may occur when there is no specific scientific question driving the analysis and in multiple regression with more than a single covariate. For example, suppose we are interested in understanding the correlates of total medical expenditures in the MEPS 2017 data, but we have not formulated any hypotheses about specific dependencies. If we test each available covariate individually and use the 0.05 threshold to select which are significant correlates of total expenditures, the probability of incorrectly rejecting the null hypothesis each time will be 0.05, but the probability of incorrectly rejecting the null hypothesis at least once could be considerably greater than 0.05. If we conduct k independent tests, the probability of at least one incorrect rejection is $1 - (1 - 0.05)^k$, which works out to 0.23 for $k = 5$ tests and to 0.40 for $k = 10$ tests.

Many different approaches have been advanced to deal with the multiple comparisons problem. The simplest and most common is to conduct each test using a more stringent criterion to reject the null hypothesis, so that the overall error rate remains at or close to 0.05. When there are very large numbers of tests, for example, in the setting of a high-dimensional genomic analysis, alternative approaches have been developed based on controlling the *false discovery rate* [e.g., 7, 8]. In other settings, awareness of the problem is a good reason to spend time developing a strong conceptual model and specifying statistical hypotheses even before you begin your analysis. If you find that you cannot avoid conducting more than a few hypothesis tests and you present individual p-values, make sure to also address the issue of multiple comparisons.

Finally, people sometimes forget that the p-value is itself a statistic; it is therefore subject to uncertainty that it inherits from the sample data. Therefore, it should not be surprising that even rigorous confirmatory studies do not always produce results that replicate prior findings, particularly when the prior p-values are based on modest sample sizes. Therefore, in analyses of datasets of any size, we recommend focusing on effect sizes and practical significance alongside statistical significance. While many academic research journals and reviewers still expect p-values to be reported, there is growing recognition of the limitations of p-values and the need for reproducibility [9].

2.5 Software and Data

R code to download data and to carry out the examples in this chapter is available at the GitHub page, https://roman-gulati.github.io/statistics-for-health-data-science/.

References

1. Andersen, R., Newman, J.F.: Societal and individual determinants of medical care utilization in the United States. The Milbank memorial fund quarterly. Health Soc. **51**, 95–124 (1973)
2. Agency for Healthcare Research and Quality: Medical expenditure panel survey (2020). http://www.ahrq.gov/research/data/meps/index.html. Accessed Feb 12 2020
3. Hayat, M.J.: Understanding statistical significance. Nurs. Res. **59**, 219–223 (2010)
4. Gelman, A., O'Rourke, K.: Discussion: difficulties in making inferences about scientific truth from distributions of published p-values. Biostatistics **15**(1), 18–23; discussion 39–45 (2014)
5. Wasserstein, R.L., Lazar, N.A.: The ASA's statement on p-values: context, process, and purpose. Am. Stat. **70**, 129–133 (2016)
6. Gelman, A., Hill, J., Yajima, M.: Why we (usually) don't have to worry about multiple comparisons (2009). arXiv:0907.2478
7. Benjamini, Y., Yekutieli, D.: False discovery rate-adjusted multiple confidence intervals for selected parameters. J. Am. Stat. Assoc. **100**, 71–81 (2005)
8. Glickman, M.E., Rao, S.R., Schultz, M.R.: False discovery rate control is a recommended alternative to Bonferroni-type adjustments in health studies. J. Clin. Epidemiol. **67**(8), 850–857 (2014)
9. Committee on Applied and Theoretical Statistics; Board on Mathematical Sciences and Their Applications Division on Engineering and Physical Sciences National Academies of Sciences Engineering and Medicine: Statistical Challenges in Assessing and Fostering the Reproducibility of Scientific Results: Summary of a Workshop. National Academies Press, Washington (2016)

Chapter 3
Regression Analysis

Abstract This chapter introduces regression analysis, the cornerstone of hypothesis-driven inquiry about health care outcomes. Regression analysis is the quantitative framework that is most commonly used to establish whether outcomes are associated with individual, community, or environmental characteristics. It quantifies the strength of relationships in conceptual models of health care utilization and costs. It provides a framework for explaining why some people incur extremely high health care expenses and why others barely cost anything. It estimates effects of health interventions. And it enables prediction of future costs and outcomes. This chapter presumes a basic knowledge of the concepts of linear regression (also known as ordinary least squares regression). We do not focus on mathematical details; rather, we present the critical ideas that form a practical foundation for regression analysis using observational health care databases.

3.1 Introduction

The basic question of how variables relate to one another is fundamental across the spectrum of health services and health outcome research. Regression analysis is a body of statistical tools and techniques that exists specifically to answer this question. Traditional regression analysis focuses on modeling the relationship between the mean of an outcome and subject characteristics. Different regression techniques are appropriate depending on the specific question of interest and the data available. In this chapter, we build a foundation for the different types of regression analyses that will be tackled in later chapters, building on standard linear regression modeling for cross-sectional data. As an example, we will study trends in overweight and obese persons in the United States, where the outcome is body mass index (BMI) and our goal is to summarize the association between mean BMI and calendar year.

Coauthored by E. Ulloa-Pérez
Department of Biostatistics, University of Washington

R. Etzioni et al., *Statistics for Health Data Science*, Springer Texts in Statistics,
https://doi.org/10.1007/978-3-030-59889-1_3

Certain outcomes and types of questions call for specialized regression techniques. If, instead of tracking the average BMI, we wish to learn how the third quartile (75th percentile) or the highest decile (90th percentile) of BMI changes over time, quantile regression would be appropriate. This type of regression is discussed in Sect. 3.10. If we are interested in tracking the proportion of the population that is overweight or obese, we would likely consider a different type of regression analysis tailored for a binary outcome, such as logistic regression; this is dealt with in Chap. 4. If we are interested in studying health care utilization outcomes (e.g., numbers of hospitalizations and outpatient visits), we would likely consider regression analysis techniques tailored to count outcomes, such as Poisson or negative binomial regression; these techniques are discussed in Chap. 5.

A prototype for regression analysis of medical expenditures is a study of the economic costs of chronic pain in the United States [1]. Here, the research question is about the link between chronic pain as assessed via survey questions and annual medical expenditures, extracted from administrative records of the survey participants. To what extent are annual medical expenditures increased for persons who report that they experience chronic pain? Since, in any given year, a fraction of the population does not use any medical care, the distribution of annual medical expenditures includes a portion of values that are zero. The rest of the values are non-zero, reflecting the expenditures for the portion of the population that did in fact access medical care that year. A specialized regression technique, discussed in Chap. 6, is needed to handle this type of mixture.

There are many other factors that may drive medical expenditures in addition to, and potentially in lockstep with, chronic pain. In the chronic pain study [1], the stated goal is to capture the "incremental costs of medical care due to pain by comparing the costs of health care of persons with chronic pain to those who do not report chronic pain, *controlling for health needs, demographic characteristics, and socioeconomic status*" (emphasis added). We discuss what is meant by "controlling for" variables in regression analysis in this chapter, but we defer the actual analysis of the incremental medical expenditures associated with a specific condition to Chap. 6, which describes methods for analyzing cost outcomes, and Chap. 8, which discusses causal inference.

Once we have clarified the research question, we select a regression model that is appropriate given the type and scale of the outcome. Here we review linear regression methods for a continuous outcome (BMI). However, the essential principles of linear regression apply across the range of models, and later chapters will build on the basic ideas presented in this one.

3.2 Trends in Body Mass Index in the United States

The National Health and Nutrition Examination Survey (NHANES) is a program of studies designed to assess nutrition and health status among children and adults in the United States [2]. The NHANES began in the early 1960s and examines a nationally representative sample of about 5000 individuals every 2 years. In addition to collecting self-reported information about nutrition and health, the NHANES also conducts physical examinations of participants and assembles a broad range of objective health measurements, including anthropometric measures and markers associated with chronic conditions like hypertension and diabetes.

The NHANES is the most authoritative source of data on overweight and obese persons in the United States, and it is the go-to resource for studies of trends in BMI over time [3]. BMI is a measure of body fat based on height and weight; it is calculated as the body mass in kilograms divided by the square of the body height in meters. The World Health Organization defines an adult with BMI between 25.0 and 29.9 as overweight and a BMI of 30.0 or higher as obese. A BMI of 18.5 to 24.9 is classified as normal or healthy weight and below 18.5 as underweight.

Many studies have been conducted of BMI trends in the United States, sounding an alarm about the obesity epidemic and its implications for chronic disease morbidity and mortality. In this chapter, we use regression analysis to study data from NHANES surveys conducted in 1999–2000 and 2015–2016 to quantify the change in BMI over this interval and how it relates to age, sex, and race/ethnicity. We focus on BMI in adults age 20–59 years since patterns of body weight and their drivers can differ markedly in younger and older persons. We briefly examine an unrestricted age range in Sect. 3.11. Although the NHANES follows a complex survey design including stratification, clustering, and weighting, these topics are postponed to Chap. 9; we do not use the survey design variables to produce the results in this chapter.

3.3 Regression Overview

There are many ways to think about regression. In essence, regression is a way of learning about mechanisms, or drivers, of an outcome. By convention, we usually use the variable X to denote the driver(s) and Y to denote the outcome. The variable X is called the *independent variable*, *covariate*, *risk factor*, *predictor*, or *feature*, and Y is the *dependent variable*, *response*, or *outcome*. We assume that it is possible to clearly identify which variables are covariates and which are outcomes, and we focus on univariate regression models which have a single outcome.

In some observational settings, it may be hard to distinguish covariate from outcome, for instance, when studying the association between depression and insomnia. Does insomnia lead to depression, or is insomnia a symptom of depression? In such settings, multivariate regression approaches which jointly model more than one outcome may be called for. In our example, Y is BMI, and X represents a list of variables: age, sex, race/ethnicity, and calendar year. We consider four distinct but connected ways of thinking about linear regression: to quantify association, to explain variability, to estimate the effect of an intervention, and to predict future outcomes. All use the same analytic framework, but they reflect different perspectives and potentially also different objectives.

3.3.1 Regression to Quantify Association

Our first perspective of regression is as a way to quantify the extent to which a covariate (X) is associated with an outcome (Y). The term "association" conveys a generic relationship observed between X and Y that may or may not be causal. This perspective zeros in on whether X is a driver of Y, even though, in observational settings, establishing an association is not the same as establishing causality. Linear regression provides a one-number summary of how the mean of Y ($E(Y)$) changes as X changes. A non-linear association can be studied by including covariates (e.g., $\log(X)$ or X^2) or by transforming the response Y (e.g., $\log(Y)$) in the regression analysis.

3.3.2 Regression to Explain Variability

This perspective focuses on understanding the variability of Y. The more specific question is: How much of the variability can be attributed to variation in values of X? Is the observed variability in Y random fluctuation, or is there something systematic to it driven by X? In the case of linear regression, we can replace the word "systematic" by "linear"; if all of the variability in Y is driven by X, then we expect the values of Y to fall on a line in the X–Y plane.

Figure 3.1 illustrates this perspective. Both panels of the figure show the same points, representing pairs of X and Y. The left panel also shows the variability of Y as deviations of the Y values from the horizontal line at the average Y value; this panel ignores any dependence of Y on X and amounts to assuming that there is no systematic component. The right panel gives more insight into how much of

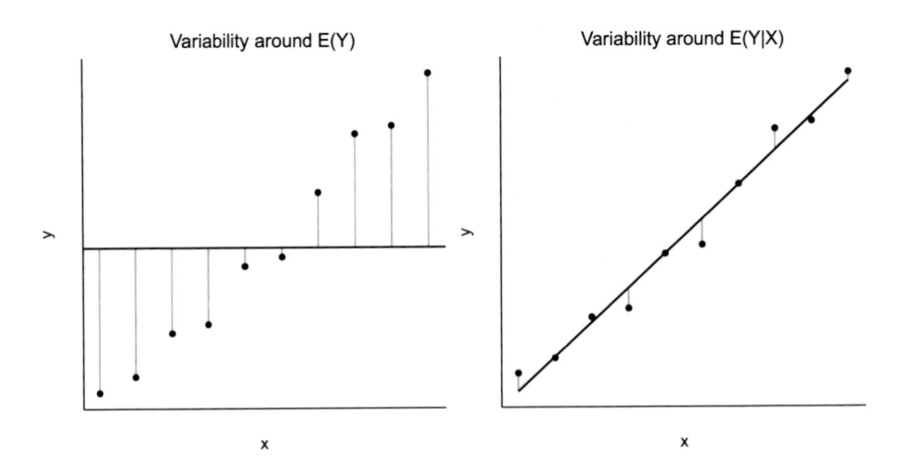

Fig. 3.1 Variability of Y values around $E(Y)$ and around $E(Y \mid X)$

the variability in Y can be explained by a linear relationship with X. It shows a line that reflects the dependence of Y on X (i.e., a positive linear association) and shows how the deviations of Y around this line are much smaller on average than the deviations of Y from the horizontal line in the left panel. We would infer from Fig. 3.1 that much of the variance of Y is explained by variation in X and there is little unexplained variance. The modest unexplained variance may be attributable to other X variables and/or to random variation in the population.

Figure 3.1 also illustrates that there is a connection between our first perspective of regression analysis, to quantify association, and this perspective, to explain variability. The figure shows that in the linear regression setting, a variable X that explains much of the variability in Y is also one that is strongly associated with Y. The converse is not always true, however; in the setting of health care utilization and costs, it is possible or even common for a variable or set of variables X to be associated with Y but not to explain much of the variability in Y.

3.3.3 Regression to Estimate the Effect of an Intervention

Like the first perspective, this one also focuses on the association between a driver X and an outcome Y, but this perspective specifically considers drivers that are interventions. An *intervention* is an activity or process designed to change outcomes, such as a new treatment to improve cancer survival or the practice of wearing seatbelts to reduce automobile fatalities.

Regression analyses of interventions typically aim to quantify causal effects. However, an association between X and Y based on observational data generally does not permit a causal interpretation; we do not control the value of the intervention (X), and we do not know why a specific subject selects their observed X value. Therefore, we cannot directly infer what would happen if we intervened and changed X. Nevertheless, there are methods designed for causal inference that build on a regression framework. We discuss this use of regression and the extensions that are needed to infer causality in Chap. 8.

3.3.4 Regression to Predict Outcomes

Our final perspective relates to the use of regression as an engine for predicting values of the response Y using information on the predictor(s) X. As an example, an insurance company trying to determine client premiums might want to use all available data on a new client to predict their expected annual medical expenditures.

The perspective of regression as a predictive engine dovetails with the growing field of predictive analytics in health care research, in which regression is only one potential analytic tool. In general, if a linear regression model is predictive of Y, then this is generally synonymous with X explaining a large portion of the observed

Table 3.1 Objectives, example questions, and associated tools when performing regression analysis

Objective	Example research question	Analytic tools and metrics
Quantify association	What is the incremental medical cost associated with obesity?	Coefficient estimation, hypothesis tests for coefficients, correlation analysis
Explain variability	Can socioeconomic factors account for variability in medical costs?	R^2, F-test
Estimate intervention effect	If we could eliminate chronic pain, how much would costs be reduced?	Causal inference techniques, propensity scores
Predict outcomes	Given patient characteristics and costs in 2011, what is the expected medical cost in 2012?	Statistical learning, predictive performance

variability in Y. As noted above, this implies that an association between Y and X exists. However, the opposite is not necessarily true. X may be strongly associated with Y, but it may only account for a minority of the observed variability in Y, and in this case, it may ultimately turn out to be a poor predictor.

In general, it is important to be clear about the objective of an analysis because this determines the type of regression analysis that may be appropriate, the specific model to fit to the data, the inferential tools used to test hypotheses, and the metrics selected to judge model adequacy. Ultimately, the objective determines the criteria for judging the quality of the model. Table 3.1 lists the four perspectives of regression analysis along with example research questions and inferential tools and metrics used to address the questions.

Clearly, these objectives are by no means mutually exclusive. On the contrary, the same regression model and the same tools can often be used for several objectives. However, while a model for quantifying association, for example, can also be used for prediction, its performance for the latter objective may be quite poor compared to a model tailored for that purpose. Similarly, a model built for prediction may not be a good model for understanding the effect of an intervention. The rest of this chapter focuses on the objectives of quantifying association and explaining variation. These objectives are very closely related and use similar tools; they mainly differ in the way model results are summarized. Chapters 8 and 10 are devoted to causal inference and predictive analyses.

3.4 An Organic View of Regression

At a very basic level, a regression model is just an organized collection of averages of outcomes within sub-populations defined by their covariate values. For a single binary or categorical covariate, regression reduces to calculating the average of the

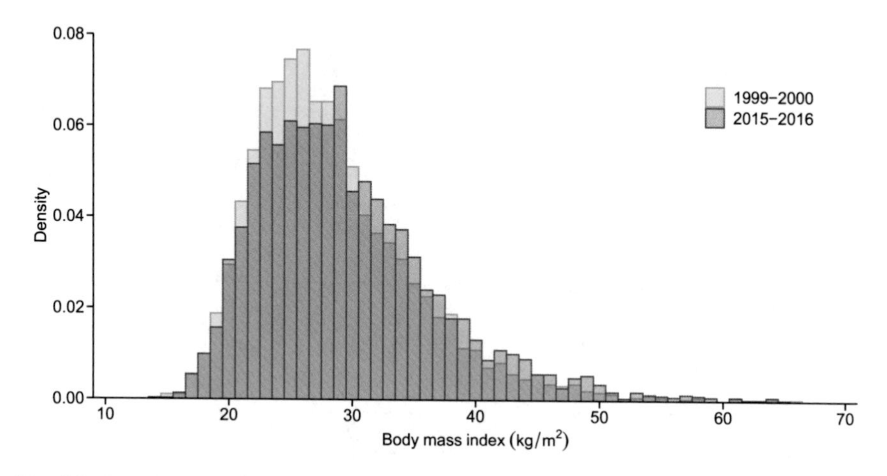

Fig. 3.2 Superimposed histograms of body mass index for persons age 20–59 years in NHANES sample data for years 1999–2000 and 2015–2016

outcome at each level of the covariate. For a continuous covariate or when there are multiple covariates, calculating the average for each sub-population separately becomes tedious. More importantly, the sample size for each sub-population may become very small, making the individual averages unreliable. Regression modeling formulates the dependence of the outcome on the covariates in a way that addresses this problem. We start with the simple case of a binary covariate and the perspective of explained variation.

Figure 3.2 shows superimposed histograms of BMI levels in 1999–2000 and 2015–2016. There is a shift toward higher BMI in 2015–2016 compared to 1999–2000. When ignoring year, average BMI is 29.1. When calculated separately, the average BMI was 28.4 in 1999–2000 and 29.6 in 2015–2016, an increase of 1.2 units.

What about the variability in BMI? When ignoring year, the variance is 49.8; this is based on subtracting the overall mean from each BMI value. How much of this variability is due to differences between years? To answer this question, we calculate the variance after subtracting the year-specific mean from each observed BMI and obtain 49.5. Thus, by considering the sub-populations defined by year, the variance is reduced from 49.8 to 49.5, a very modest reduction of $(49.8 - 49.5)/49.8 = 0.7\%$. This result suggests that less than 1% of the variability in BMI levels is attributable to calendar year. Indeed, many factors are involved in explaining population variability in BMI [3]. The fact that year explains only a small minority of the variability in BMI does not, however, imply that BMI and calendar year are not associated. In fact, we will show that there is a statistically significant increase in BMI over time.

The distribution of BMI levels can also be calculated for sub-populations defined by variables with more than two categories, such as age. Figure 3.3 shows a scatterplot of age versus BMI, with line segments indicating average BMI levels

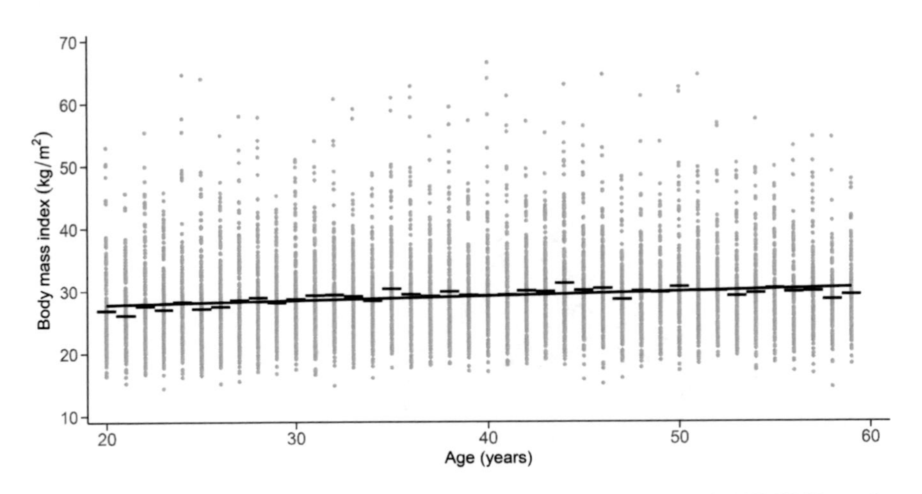

Fig. 3.3 Individual and average body mass index for persons age 20–59 years in NHANES sample data for years 1999–2000 and 2015–2016 and a fitted regression line

for each single-age sub-population. Several important properties of the data are apparent. First, average BMI levels in the sub-populations show small fluctuations from one age to the next, probably due to the small sample size within each sub-population (compared to the total sample size). Second, the average BMI tends to increase with age. Third, a straight line reasonably approximates the increasing average BMI with age. This third property motivates using the line to characterize how the average BMI changes across sub-populations defined by age. This smooths out the fluctuations due to small sample sizes and more simply represents the relationship between age and BMI.

Both smoothing and simplicity are important goals when the covariate X takes many values or there are several covariates. Table 3.2 compares average BMI calculated for each age directly to those obtained by the regression line (REG) in Fig. 3.3:

$$\text{Mean BMI} = 26.37 + 0.07 \times \text{AGE}.$$

As the table shows, the differences are relatively small, and it is much simpler to cite the regression equation to describe the relationship between age and BMI than to provide a detailed listing of averages.

The decision to replace the list of averages with a straight line is often not justified, however. Whether and when to use linear regression bring us to a closer examination of the model and its assumptions.

Table 3.2 Average body mass index for persons age 20–59 years in NHANES sample data for years 1999–2000 and 2015–2016 and values from a regression line (REG)

AGE	BMI	REG	AGE	BMI	REG	AGE	BMI	REG	AGE	BMI	REG
20	26.9	27.8	30	28.7	28.5	40	29.2	29.2	50	30.6	29.9
21	26.1	27.8	31	29.3	28.5	41	29.3	29.2	51	29.9	29.9
22	27.6	27.9	32	29.4	28.6	42	30.0	29.3	52	29.9	30.0
23	27.0	28.0	33	29.1	28.7	43	29.8	29.4	53	29.1	30.1
24	28.2	28.0	34	28.4	28.7	44	31.2	29.4	54	29.6	30.1
25	27.1	28.1	35	30.3	28.8	45	30.0	29.5	55	30.3	30.2
26	27.5	28.2	36	29.4	28.9	46	30.3	29.6	56	29.7	30.3
27	28.5	28.3	37	29.1	29.0	47	28.6	29.6	57	29.8	30.3
28	28.9	28.3	38	29.9	29.0	48	29.9	29.7	58	28.5	30.4
29	28.1	28.4	39	29.3	29.1	49	29.7	29.8	59	29.3	30.5

3.5 The Linear Regression Equation and Its Assumptions

Regardless of whether the focus is on modeling the mean of Y, explaining the variance of Y, estimating the effect of an intervention on Y, or predicting Y, the central expression of a linear regression analysis is the well-known formula for how Y depends on a set of k covariates $X_1, \ldots, X_k$:

$$E(Y \mid X_1, \ldots, X_k) = \beta_0 + \beta_1 X_1 + \cdots + \beta_k X_k.$$

The expression on the left, $E(Y \mid X_1, \ldots, X_k)$, indicates the mean of the outcome Y (e.g., BMI) in the sub-population defined by specific values for the covariates $X_1, \ldots, X_k$ (e.g., age, sex, race/ethnicity, and calendar year).The resulting regression model specifies that this depends on a linear combination of the values of the covariates.

The assumption of linearity is not trivial, and it rarely holds in observational datasets; at best, it is an approximation for how the actual mean varies across sub-populations. The linearity assumption specifies that a one-unit increase in the covariate X_1 will result in an increase of β_1 units of the mean of Y *regardless of the initial value of* X_1 *and given any set of values for the other covariates* $X_2, \ldots, X_k$. A similar interpretation applies for all the other covariates. Thus if, for example, X_1 is an indicator for year 2015–2016 with coefficient $\beta_1 = 1.6$, the model states that the average BMI increases by 1.6 units between 1999–2000 and 2015–2016 for non-Hispanic white men age 24 years, for African American women age 57 years, and so on, for all possible combinations of age, sex, and race/ethnicity.

The linear model means that the individual X values combine in an additive way to yield the mean of Y. Even if transformations of X, such as polynomials (e.g., X^2) or other non-linear functions (e.g., $\log(X)$), are added to the list of covariates, the model is still considered a linear model so long as these terms enter additively into the regression equation. The objective is to estimate the coefficients $\beta_1, \ldots, \beta_k$ that quantify the relationships between the Xs and Y.

The coefficient of a given covariate, say β_2, quantifies the association between X_2 and Y when all other Xs are held constant. The form of the linear regression model (in particular, the additive effects of the covariates) implies that the specific values of the other Xs do not matter; β_2 is the change in Y associated with a one-unit change in X_2 regardless of the values of the other Xs. In this way, we isolate the relationship between X_2 and Y, and we say that we are *adjusting* or *controlling for* the other Xs. In other words, β_2 compares the mean of Y in two sub-populations that differ only in the value of X_2.

In practice, individuals in a sub-population rarely have identical values for the response variable. For example, we do not expect that all non-Hispanic white men aged 34 to have exactly the same BMI, and we would be surprised if they did. To reflect this, we can index individuals by the letter i and write Y_i as the response for subject i and $X_{i1}, \ldots, X_{ik}$ as the covariates. The model for individual i is then:

$$Y_i = \beta_0 + \beta_1 X_{i1} + \cdots + \beta_k X_{ik} + \epsilon_i.$$

The E on the left-hand side of the previous equation that was used to indicate the mean (or *expected value*) of a sub-population is omitted, and a new term ϵ_i is added to the right-hand side to reflect a subject-specific deviation from the sub-population mean $\beta_0 + \beta_1 X_{i1} + \cdots + \beta_k X_{ik}$. We can think of the sub-population mean as the systematic part of the model and ϵ_i as the random part. In principle, a regression model performs well if the systematic part accounts for a sizeable portion of the variability. We discuss criteria for a "good" model in Sect. 3.9.

In addition to the assumed linearity and additivity for the systematic part, three key assumptions underpin the random term ϵ_i: (1) the random terms follow a normal distribution with mean zero, (2) this normal distribution has the same variance in all sub-populations, and (3) the random parts of all observations are independent, implying that the observed Y from one individual is independent of the others. These three assumptions are not actually needed to validly fit the regression model. So long as the systematic part is correctly specified, the estimates of the βs are valid and unbiased, regardless of whether assumptions (1)–(3) are satisfied. But standard errors for the β estimates are based on assumptions about the random part, and if these don't hold, the standard errors may not be valid and may ultimately generate incorrect confidence intervals, p-values, and inferences.

3.6 Linear Regression Estimation and Interpretation

3.6.1 Estimation of the Regression Coefficients

There are two main methods for estimating the βs: *least squares* and *maximum likelihood*. Each method amounts to solving an optimization problem.

In least squares, the problem is to identify the βs that minimize the sum of the squared differences between the responses Y and the systematic part of the regression equation, $\beta_0 + \beta_1 X_1 + \cdots + \beta_k X_k$, which is a straight line. Varying the βs moves this line around, and the optimal solution is given by those βs corresponding to the regression line that is "closest" to the observed responses. Squared differences are a convenient measure of closeness as they make all the differences positive. Other measures, such as absolute differences, can be harder to work with mathematically.

Figure 3.1 demonstrates the least squares approach. As noted above, the two panels present different straight lines and show corresponding vertical differences between the responses and the lines. The sum of squared differences is clearly smaller for the line in the right panel, so this line is better in terms of total squared differences. Of course, there are many more lines to consider, but it turns out that finding the least squares line is a simple computational task, and the line in the right panel is indeed the regression line—the line minimizing the sum of the squared differences between model and data. Note that the method does not use any of the assumptions regarding the random part of the regression equation; instead, it fits the regression line using only the systematic part.

In maximum likelihood, we exploit the random part of the model. Maximum likelihood tries to determine the line $\beta_0 + \beta_1 X_1 + \cdots + \beta_k X_k$ that is most plausible or most likely to have generated the observed Y values. Thinking about the observed Ys as fixed (since they have already been observed), we vary the βs until we find values that maximize the probability of observing those Ys under those βs. Since the probability of observing any specific value of Y depends on the distribution of Y, maximum likelihood depends on the assumptions regarding the random part of the model.

Maximum likelihood requires that we know more about the data than least squares—we cannot perform maximum likelihood without specifying the distribution of the random term. While this may seem like a liability, what we gain in return (if our specification is correct) is an assurance of efficiency—the βs are the most precise available under the specified linear model—and, if the systematic part is also correct, valid inference, including correct confidence intervals and p-values.

When the random part is normally distributed, the least squares estimates are identical to the maximum likelihood estimates. Because of the mathematics of the normal distribution, finding the line that minimizes the sum of squared differences between the Ys and the regression line is the same as finding the line that maximizes the probability of the observed Ys. Thus, in this case, the least squares approach inherits all of the favorable properties of the maximum likelihood approach. In all other cases, including the settings discussed in later chapters, we will use maximum likelihood to accommodate the non-normal distribution of the Ys.

3.6.2 Interpretation of the Regression Coefficients

Table 3.3 provides the results from fitting a linear regression model to NHANES data for persons age 20–59 years in 1999–2000 and 2015–2016. The outcome is BMI, and the main question is how this outcome has changed over time. We have two time points, and the regression equation includes a binary variable SEX (with reference level male), a categorical variable RACE (with reference level non-Hispanic white) coded as a set of dummy variables, a binary variable AGE (with reference level $\leq$50 years), and a binary variable YEAR (with reference level 1999–2000). Although we will show that assumptions of normality and constant variance are likely not satisfied for this regression model, we use it here to illustrate interpretation of the regression coefficients that comprise the systematic part of the model.

The intercept represents mean BMI at the reference level for all variables. Thus, the regression analysis estimates that the mean BMI for non-Hispanic white men age $\leq$50 years in 1999–2000 was 26.97.

The coefficient for YEAR is 1.54, meaning that the average BMI increased by 1.54 units from the 1999–2000 survey to the 2015–2016 survey. The estimated coefficient is the same within each sub-population defined by the other covariates. That the estimate, 1.54, is interpreted as a difference (between later and earlier calendar years) and that this difference is the same across all sub-populations defined by the other covariates are consequences of the model assumptions of additivity and linearity.

The standard errors (SEs) reflect uncertainty in the estimated regression coefficients. This uncertainty is often reported as 95% confidence intervals by adding and subtracting scaled SEs from the estimates. The scaling factor is determined by the distribution of the coefficient estimates. These estimates are typically assumed to be normally distributed, but this is only true if the response Y is normal or the sample size is relatively large [4], as is the case with the NHANES dataset. The 95% confidence interval for the increase in BMI during the 15 years examined is $1.54 \pm 1.96 \times 0.18$, or 1.19 to 1.89.

In the preceding example, an individual's age was coded as a binary variable. Table 3.4 shows the fitted regression model if age is coded as a continuous variable

Table 3.3 Change in body mass index between 1999–2000 and 2015–2016 for persons age 20–59 years in NHANES sample data controlling for categorical age, sex, and race/ethnicity

Variable	Coefficient	SE	*P*-value
Intercept	26.97	0.20	<0.001
SEX = Female	1.07	0.17	<0.001
RACE = Non-Hispanic black	1.95	0.24	<0.001
RACE = Mexican American	1.38	0.23	<0.001
RACE = Other Hispanic	0.78	0.31	0.01
RACE = Other/Mixed	−2.39	0.30	<0.001
AGE = >50	0.65	0.21	0.002
YEAR = 2015–2016	1.54	0.18	<0.001

Table 3.4 Change in body mass index between 1999–2000 and 2015–2016 for persons age 20–59 years in NHANES sample data controlling for continuous age and categorical sex and race/ethnicity

Variable	Coefficient	SE	*P*-value
Intercept	24.51	0.35	<0.001
SEX = Female	1.10	0.17	<0.001
RACE = Non-Hispanic black	1.93	0.24	<0.001
RACE = Mexican American	1.44	0.23	<0.001
RACE = Other Hispanic	0.79	0.31	<0.01
RACE = Other/mixed	−2.35	0.30	<0.001
AGE	0.07	0.01	<0.001
YEAR = 2015–2016	1.47	0.18	<0.001

Table 3.5 Analytic considerations for coding covariates in a regression equation

Type of covariate	Questions
Continuous	Is linearity appropriate?
	What does zero mean?
	Should it be centered and/or scaled for interpretability?
Unordered categorical	What is the reference level?
	Should categories be combined?
Ordered categorical	Should it be recoded as continuous or unordered?
	Should it be dichotomized?

instead. The model estimates a slightly smaller increase in mean BMI over time, about 1.47 units.

The regression intercept still represents mean BMI at the reference level for all categorical variables and, now that a continuous variable is included, when that variable is equal to zero. Because mean BMI at age 0 years may be awkward and in other examples even nonsensical, it is often helpful to center the continuous variable, for example, by subtracting the median age (38 years in this sample). Then, the intercept represents mean BMI for non-Hispanic white men age 38 years in 1999–2000. Scaling continuous variables may also help with interpretation. For example, dividing age by 10 means that a one-unit increase in the rescaled age variable corresponds to a 10-year increase in age, which is associated with an increase of 0.7 units in mean BMI in this example.

For categorical or factor covariates, consideration should be given to the choice of reference level. The reference level should be meaningful for the analysis and adequately represented in the sample. For race/ethnicity in this example, we used non-Hispanic white as the reference level. Ordered categorical variables can sometimes be specified as continuous variables (e.g., by replacing household income brackets by their midpoints), but this will impose strict constraints that may not match the data (linear dependence on household brackets). Table 3.5 summarizes some important analytic considerations and principles when incorporating different types of variables in the regression equation.

3.6.3 Confounding

It is tempting to interpret the coefficient of a covariate as its causal effect on the outcome, meaning that changing the value of that covariate by one unit will result in a change of the outcome by the corresponding β coefficient. However, in observational data the covariate of interest is often associated with other covariates that vary together to affect the outcome. This phenomenon, called confounding, is an unavoidable problem whenever observational data are analyzed. Formally, we define a covariate Z as being a *confounder* of the association between X and Y if Z affects both X and Y.

Confounding is a primary reason for why we must be very cautious when making causal inferences from observational data and why we always have to question whether there may be other explanations for any associations identified between a covariate and the outcome. Chapter 8 provides a detailed treatment of confounding and causal inference; here, we briefly explain the issue in terms of the mechanics of regression analysis with multiple covariates.

For clarity, suppose we are interested in the association between an outcome Y and a covariate X. For example, Y may be BMI and X may be a binary indicator of regular physical exercise (PE), with $X = 1$ if yes and $X = 0$ if no. In the NHANES sample data from 2015–2016, a question about weekly recreational exercise asked: "In a typical week do you do any vigorous-intensity sports, fitness, or recreational activities that cause large increases in breathing or heart rate like running or basketball for at least 10 min continuously?" We use the response to this question as our PE variable.

It is well known that, as we age, we become less active and BMI tends to increase; thus AGE could be reasonably considered to be a confounder in our analysis because it affects both BMI and PE. In the NHANES sample data, again restricted to ages 20–59 years, there is a significant negative correlation between AGE and PE and, as previously shown, a significant positive correlation between AGE and BMI.

Running a simple linear regression of BMI on PE, we unsurprisingly find that average BMI is significantly lower for individuals who exercise, with the estimated coefficient of PE equal to -2.15. If we intervene and convince all inactive individuals to engage in regular physical exercise, is it reasonable to expect a reduction of 2.15 units in average BMI?

The problem with interpreting this association as a causal relationship is that AGE is lurking in the shadows. As the PE indicator changes from 0 to 1, the corresponding sub-population becomes younger; the PE variable and the AGE variable change together. Thus, in the simple linear regression with just PE as the lone covariate, the estimated association between BMI and PE is boosted by the (lurking) association between AGE and PE. When we include both PE and AGE in the model, the coefficient of PE is still negative and significant, but it is reduced in magnitude to -1.88. The boost from the implicit effect of the younger sub-population is gone because the effect of PE is estimated keeping age constant. When we interpret the coefficient of PE, we are now assessing only the effect of PE on

BMI, adjusting or controlling for the effect of AGE. This explanation assumes that the linear model is correct, and there are likely other confounders of the BMI-PE association, making causal interpretation on the basis of these few covariates a bit of a stretch. Still, this example serves to illustrate the mechanics of confounder adjustment in multiple regression.

In observational studies, associations of interest are almost always subject to confounding, sometimes by multiple variables. We provide more detail and discussion of causal inference in the presence of confounding in Chap. 8.

3.6.4 Moderation or Interaction

In the previous sections, an increase in mean BMI over time was assumed to be the same in all sub-populations. But is the change in mean BMI over time indeed the same for younger as for older persons? Is it the same for all racial/ethnic groups? This question brings us to the concept of *effect modification*, also called *moderation* or *interaction*.

Effect modification occurs when the association between a covariate X and an outcome Y differs according to the levels of another covariate (Z). We say that covariate Z *modifies* or *moderates* the association between X and Y. In the case where X is YEAR and Z is (categorical) AGE, we say that AGE modifies the association between YEAR and BMI if the change in BMI over time differs for younger versus older persons. There are at least two ways to learn about whether the association between YEAR and BMI is modified by AGE:

1. Fit two separate regression models corresponding to the two levels of AGE. In our example, this would yield one analysis for persons age $\leq$50 years and another analysis for persons age $>$50 years.
2. Fit a single regression model, but include an interaction term (i.e., the product of YEAR and AGE) in the linear model that already includes these covariates.

The first approach provides separate estimates of the association between X and Y within each subgroup defined by the levels of Z. However, it also provides separate estimates of the regression coefficients for all other covariates in the model. Not only is this approach potentially inefficient, it also does not provide a formal mechanism for testing whether the association between X and Y differs across the levels of Z.

Equation (3.1) shows the regression equation for the second approach:

$$E(Y) = \beta_0 + \beta_1 \text{YEAR} + \beta_2 \text{AGE} + \beta_3 \text{AGE} \times \text{YEAR}. \tag{3.1}$$

The interaction term is non-zero when both AGE and YEAR are equal to 1. It therefore contributes to $E(Y)$ only for the older age group in 2015–2016. This means that, when we estimate the change in mean BMI from 1999–2000 to 2015–2016, we end up with a different estimate for older than for younger persons.

Table 3.6 Change in body mass index between 1999–2000 and 2015–2016 for persons age 20–59 years in NHANES sample data controlling for categorical age, sex, race/ethnicity, and age-year interaction

Variable	Coefficient	SE	*P*-value
Intercept	26.92	0.20	<0.001
SEX = Female	1.07	0.17	<0.001
RACE = Non-Hispanic black	1.96	0.24	<0.001
RACE = Mexican American	1.39	0.23	<0.001
RACE = Other Hispanic	0.79	0.31	0.01
RACE = Other/mixed	−2.40	0.30	<0.001
AGE = >50	0.95	0.34	0.006
YEAR = 2015–2016	1.64	0.20	<0.001
AGE-YEAR interaction	−0.49	0.44	0.3

Specifically, the change for younger persons is given by β_1, and the change for older persons is given by $\beta_1 + \beta_3$. Symmetrically, when we estimate the difference in mean BMI for older versus younger persons, we end up with a different estimate for 1999–2000 (β_2) than for 2015–2016 ($\beta_2 + \beta_3$). The same idea also applies when YEAR is continuous, in which case the interaction term implies a different slope of the corresponding regression line for older versus younger persons.

Table 3.6 repeats the analysis in Table 3.3 but adds an interaction between AGE and YEAR. The interaction term is negative; the estimated change in BMI from 1999–2000 to 2015–2016 is less for older than for younger individuals. The global change over the 15-year period of 1.54 units presented in Table 3.3 that does not include an interaction term is replaced here with a change of 1.64 units for younger and $1.64 - 0.49 = 1.15$ units for older individuals.

Because the model implies that the change in mean BMI depends on AGE, we cannot interpret the coefficient of the YEAR variable as a stand-alone estimate of the change in mean BMI over time. In general, when there is an interaction term in the model, the *main effects* (i.e., the coefficients of the covariates that go into the interaction) cannot be interpreted by themselves without qualification. To understand why, recall that the coefficient of a single variable X is interpreted as the expected change in Y corresponding to a unit change in X *holding values for all the other covariates in the model constant.* In the model of BMI with an AGE-YEAR interaction, we cannot change the values of AGE or YEAR by one unit while holding the interaction term (product of AGE and YEAR) fixed. Therefore, we cannot interpret the coefficients of AGE and YEAR in the standard manner. This is an important point to remember in general in regression analysis; interpretation of coefficients is *conditional*, and if we cannot conceive of changing one covariate in isolation while holding the others constant, then we may have to re-think our model or its interpretation.

Figure 3.4 shows distributions of BMI levels using centered, stacked dots representing binned observations with lines connecting means for the two survey years within each age, sex, and race/ethnicity stratum. A simple linear model without any interaction term assumes that all the slopes are equal, so that the effect of year is the same in all sub-populations. The figure shows some deviation from that assumption, suggesting that changes in BMI levels over time may not be the same for all sub-populations.

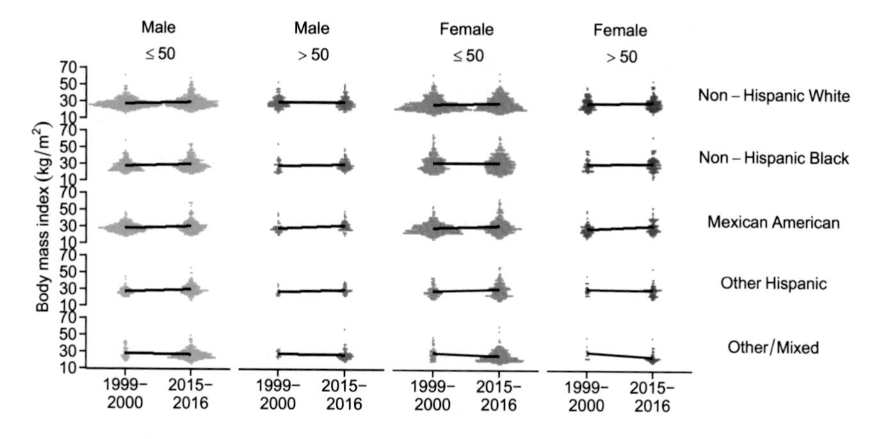

Fig. 3.4 Dotplots and lines showing mean change in body mass index between 1999–2000 and 2015–2016 for persons age 20–59 years in NHANES sample data by age, sex, and race/ethnicity

3.7 Model Selection and Hypothesis Testing

Several models for mean BMI were fit in the previous section, and many other models could be considered. How should we choose the final model? Then, once a final model is selected, how do we evaluate it and draw valid inferences?

There is a direct line from the objective of the analysis to the final model selected and the evaluation of its goodness. If the objective is to test a pre-specified scientific hypothesis, decisions about which variables to include are appropriately guided by a conceptual model and should be made before examining the data. If this is not possible, or if the analyst's intent is to use the data to identify variables that are predictive, classical inference and hypothesis testing based on the fitted model are not warranted and can be seriously biased.

When we are addressing pre-specified hypotheses, the significance of a single covariate may be evaluated using the *Wald test* of the null hypothesis that a given coefficient (β) is different from zero [5]. In the BMI example, the coefficient of SEX is highly significant (p-value <0.001) in all regressions (Tables 3.3, 3.4, 3.5, and 3.6), but the coefficient of the interaction between AGE and YEAR is not significant at the conventional 5% level (Table 3.6). These p-values are based on the ratio of the estimated coefficient to its standard error. They are obtained by comparing this ratio to the quantiles of a normal distribution, thus assuming that the estimated coefficients are normally distributed. This is true if the response Y is normal or the sample size is large [4].

To evaluate the significance of two or more coefficients, we can employ the *likelihood ratio test* [5], a powerful approach for many statistical testing problems. The test evaluates the hypothesis that at least one of the coefficients is different from zero. In the BMI example, the RACE variable is a categorical variable with four coefficients for the non-reference levels, so testing whether there is an association between BMI and RACE amounts to testing whether the coefficient for any non-reference level is different from zero. Even though the RACE variable is converted to four dummy variables, these represent a single construct (RACE) and should be tested together.

The likelihood ratio test is equivalent to comparing a restricted regression model ($M_{\text{restricted}}$), in which all of these coefficients are set to zero (equivalently, fitting a new model without the variable RACE), and a full model (M_{full}), in which these coefficients are allowed to take on (theoretically) any value. These two models are said to be nested because one is a restricted version of the other. The test compares the likelihood (L) under the full model to that under the restricted model.

Recall that the likelihood is the probability of the data that was observed under the postulated model and the β coefficients were chosen in order to maximize this probability. If we add more variables to the regression model (e.g., adding RACE or adding a new interaction term), we provide more explanatory power and the likelihood will typically increase. The likelihood ratio test is a way of determining whether adding RACE to the model adds more explanatory power than would be expected by chance. Note that the test is appropriate only when comparing two nested models, that is, when the restricted model can be obtained by setting one or more of the coefficients in the full model to zero.

The likelihood ratio test for linear regression with a normally distributed error term is equivalent to an F-test that compares the explained variation of the full and restricted models. Specifically, it compares the residual or unexplained variance in the full model, $\text{Var}_{\text{res}}(M_{\text{full}})$, to that in the restricted model, $\text{Var}_{\text{res}}(M_{\text{restricted}})$.[1] Essentially, it tests whether this unexplained variance is significantly reduced when comparing the full model with the restricted model.

Certain conditions are needed for these tests to be valid. The F-test relies on the least squares formulation of the regression problem and does not assume a distribution for the response Y. In contrast, the likelihood ratio test specifies a distribution for the response—a normal distribution in the case of linear regression. Thus, the F-test relies on the validity of the least squares approach, while the likelihood ratio test relies, in addition, on the validity of the assumed distribution. Applying either test in our BMI example, we find that the association between BMI and RACE is highly significant (p-value <0.001).

In some settings, we may be interested in comparing models that are not nested, e.g., when selecting the final model. For example, we may want to compare models that include log(AGE) instead of AGE or to compare a categorical coding of AGE versus a continuous coding of AGE. Of course, if we compare a model with many covariates to a model with only few, the former may perform better simply because it is more flexible and carries more explanatory power. To even the playing field when comparing less versus more flexible models, a common approach is to penalize the

[1]Many textbooks present this test in terms of the residual sum of squares (RSS) instead of the variance as used here. These are equivalent approaches since $\text{RSS} = (n-1) \times \text{Var}_{\text{res}}$, where n is the number of observations in the data.

measured performance by the number of parameters used; as the model becomes more flexible, the penalty goes up. Two likelihood-based statistics that take this approach are the Akaike Information Criterion (AIC) and the Bayesian Information Criterion (BIC). These are scaled versions of the negative (maximized) likelihood for a given model (M), but each imposes a penalty for including more variables in the model. Specifically, these statistics are defined as:[2]

$$\text{AIC} = -2\log[L(M)] + 2k$$
$$\text{BIC} = -2\log[L(M)] + k\log(n).$$

Here, k denotes the number of parameters in the model (e.g., in a linear model, k is equal to the number of βs plus 1 for σ^2, the variance of the residuals, which is also estimated). As the model becomes more complex and the likelihood increases, the first term decreases, but the second term increases. The model that minimizes the sum of the two terms is preferred. Thus, the goal is to find the model that minimizes the AIC (or BIC). The two statistics are similar, but the BIC imposes a more severe penalty for model complexity, so it may select simpler, more parsimonious models than the AIC in certain cases.

Table 3.7 shows the number of parameters, log likelihood, AIC, and BIC for the regression models with age coded as a categorical or as a continuous variable with and without the AGE-YEAR interaction term.

Both the AIC and BIC are smallest for the model with age coded as a continuous variable without the AGE–YEAR interaction term. Consequently, this model should be preferred among the four. Whether this is a "good" model, however, depends on how it will be used. This topic is taken up in Sect. 3.9.

One important thing to remember is that although the likelihood depends on the random part of the model, the model selection methods compare only the systematic part of the model, and not other aspects like the distribution of the response. In particular, all models that are compared must use the same response variable, so a model with BMI coded as continuous cannot be compared to a model with BMI coded as a binary response or a model that uses a transformation

Table 3.7 Summary statistics for four linear regression models of body mass index for persons age 20–59 years in NHANES sample data for 1999–2000 and 2015–2016

Age	Interaction	Parameters	Log likelihood	AIC	BIC
Categorical	No	9	−21585.4	43188.9	43249.8
Continuous	No	9	−21551.1	43120.2	43181.2
Categorical	Yes	10	−21584.8	43189.7	43257.4
Continuous	Yes	10	−21551.1	43122.2	43189.9

[2]Here and everywhere else in this text, the "log" function refers to the natural logarithm, which is sometimes denoted "ln."

of BMI, such as log(BMI). Transformations are allowed only for the covariates (Xs). The models must also be based on the same set of observations. This is a point that is sometimes overlooked, particularly as some estimation software quietly drops observations with missing values for covariates, which may lead to different numbers of observations in models with different sets of covariates.

3.8 Checking Assumptions About the Random Part

The previous section focused on selecting and testing hypotheses about the systematic part of the model. This section discusses the assumptions underlying the random part. Checking whether these assumptions are satisfied is important because their violation can lead to invalid inference, including incorrect confidence intervals and biased p-values.

Recall the three basic assumptions regarding the residuals: (1) that they have a normal distribution, (2) that their variance is similar in all sub-populations (i.e., the variance does not depend on the Xs), and (3) that they are independent. We discuss graphical checks for the first two. The third assumption is usually verified on a case-by-case basis by scrutinizing whether the sample collection imposed dependencies between individuals, such as repeated measurements or observations that were clustered together (e.g., patients treated in the same hospital).

Figure 3.5 shows diagnostic plots to assess the normality and constant variance assumptions in the BMI example. The left panel shows a *quantile-quantile* or *QQ-normal* plot, where the empirical quantiles of the model residuals are plotted against the theoretical quantiles expected under a normal model. When the normality assumption holds, the QQ-normal plot shows a linear trend. Because the quantiles of

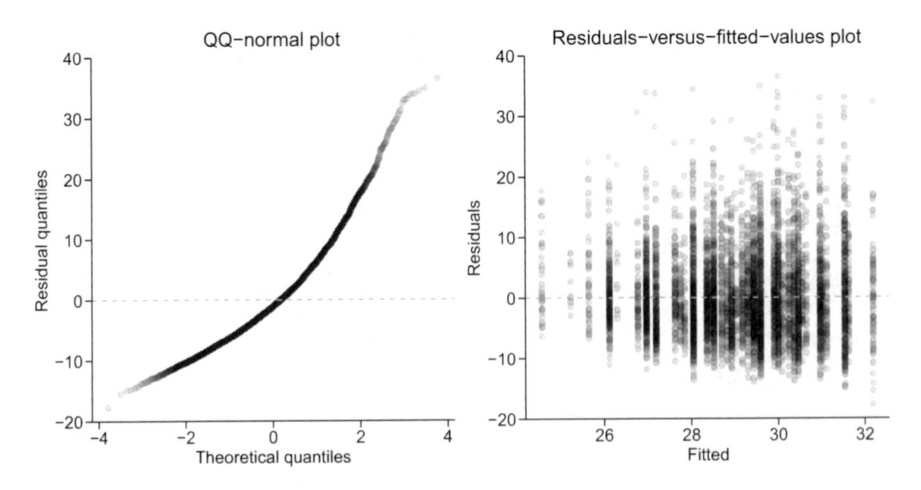

Fig. 3.5 QQ-normal and residuals-versus-fitted-values plots for the linear regression in Table 3.3

the model residuals are not linearly related to the theoretical quantiles from a normal distribution, the assumption of normality is suspect for this model. The right panel shows a scatterplot of residuals versus fitted values. Because the variance of the residuals increases for larger fitted values, the assumption of constant variance also appears to be violated in this model. Issues with non-normality diminish in large samples [4], but nonconstant variance may still impact the validity of hypothesis tests and p-values.

Standard errors for the βs also assume that the observations are independent. This independence may not hold for clustered observations (e.g., body mass measurements taken from multiple members of a household) or observations that are taken close together in space or time (e.g., income measurements from a shared census tract). When observations are not independent, the regression modeling approach can be extended to accommodate dependence even when the structure of the dependence is not known. (See Gelman and Hill [6] for a thorough treatment of regression analysis in the setting of correlated outcomes.) In general, misspecification of the model (e.g., incorrectly assuming an association is linear or that observations are independent) and omission of key covariates constitute the greatest threats to valid inference and prediction from a regression model.

3.9 Do I Have a Good Model? Goodness of Fit and Model Adequacy

The question of whether a model is "good" is tightly bound to the objective of the analysis. To be sure, each of the objectives identified in this chapter requires that the model be correctly specified. Yet different criteria emerge for evaluating model adequacy depending on how the model will be used.

In a hypothesis-driven analysis, there is a well-formed question that translates into a statistical hypothesis test, such as whether there is an increase in BMI over time. So long as the assumptions for validity of the test are satisfied, we can feel comfortable that we have a "good" model. If, for example, we use the Wald test to address whether average BMI is higher in 2015–2016 than in 1999–2000, then the relevant coefficient estimate should be normally distributed with true standard error equal to that corresponding to a standard linear regression model. Even if the data are not normal, the coefficient estimate may be normally distributed if the sample size is sufficiently large.

A popular measure that is often cited as a measure of the goodness of a regression model is the coefficient of determination (R^2), which quantifies the variance attributable to the model. For example, $R^2 = 0.70$ means that 70% of the variance in Y is due to (its dependence on) X in the data. R^2 measures the proportion of explained variation in the data, not in the population, and always increases when new covariates are added to the model. An *adjusted* R^2 (R^2_{adj}) is used to correct for this and is generally preferred. If explaining variability is the primary objective, then ideally R^2 or its adjusted version should be high. This can occur even when the regression assumptions are not all met. Conversely, a linear regression model may be perfectly satisfied, but R^2 may be quite low. For the model in Table 3.4, R^2 and R^2_{adj} are 4.8% and 4.7%, respectively. Thus, AGE, SEX, RACE, and YEAR explain approximately 5% of the variability in BMI values; such low R^2 values are typical in observational studies. In this hypothesis-driven analysis, however, the objective is to evaluate an association (between AGE and YEAR), so, as noted above, the validity of the assumptions underlying the hypothesis test is paramount. And if we want to ascribe a causal interpretation to our inferences, then the assumptions necessary for causal inference must be satisfied; these are addressed in detail in Chap. 8.

While the absolute level of R^2 is meaningful, the likelihood-based statistics including the AIC and BIC can only be used to compare models; their absolute values are not indicative of model adequacy or quality. The likelihood ratio test and the F-test can only compare nested models, and the F-test is similarly limited in that it is a comparative statistic. In fact, none of the standard tests or established summaries used in regression analysis are able to assess a model's fitness for purpose.

When prediction is the goal, accuracy of the predictions is the ultimate criterion for evaluating model adequacy. Predictive accuracy is typically summarized by the average squared prediction error (observed minus predicted values), but other summaries may be used in practice, particularly in the case of binary responses. Some considerations should be kept in mind when assessing adequacy of a prediction model. First, it may be difficult to identify a specific threshold for the predictive accuracy that reflects an adequately "good" model. Indeed, in many settings, comparisons of measures of predictive accuracy are used to judge relative rather than absolute performance of models. Second, models chosen on the basis of predictive accuracy may not be informative about the mechanistic process that generated the data. Such models are designed to predict, rather than to explain, the data. Finally, if a model is chosen on the basis of its predictive performance, then hypothesis testing of specific model estimates or coefficients is not advised; making well-founded statistical inferences on the basis of data-adaptive predictive models is still an evolving field [7–9].

If the objective of an analysis is purely to predict the response, then the models available extend far beyond regression analysis and include methods from the fields of statistical and machine learning. These methods forego any distributional assumptions, easily incorporate non-linearities, and can accommodate thousands of predictor variables. But there are also additional considerations. A model developed using one dataset may appear to have good predictive performance in that dataset (sometimes called *internal validity*) but perform poorly in another dataset (*external validity*). This occurs when the model is overfit to the training dataset, possibly because a large number of explanatory variables were included with little or no scientific rationale. For this reason, model selection is generally based on predictive performance in a cross-validation setting, and models are judged on the basis of their predictive accuracy in a validation dataset. We discuss these methods, their implementation, and limitations in Chap. 10.

3.10 Quantile Regression

In Sect. 3.4, we conceptualized a regression model as an organized collection of average outcomes across sub-populations defined by their covariate values. In some settings, other summaries are more informative about the outcome distribution than the mean. For example, we might prefer the median when the outcome is right skewed or multimodal. Or we might focus on a high percentile if we want to understand what drives high values of the outcome—for example, if we seek to investigate factors associated with people being in the highest decile of medical expenditures. We might even be interested in modeling summaries that tell us about the variability of the outcome rather than its mean.

As an example, suppose we are interested in the first and third quartiles (i.e., the 25th and 75th percentiles) of BMI for different ages. This might be motivated by questions about whether the variability in BMI grows or shrinks with age; the difference between these two quartiles (inter-quartile range) is a common measure of variability.

Figure 3.6 shows the fitted values from a *quantile regression* fit to the first and third quartiles of BMI with age as a covariate. The fitted model suggests that if linearity holds, then the inter-quartile range is approximately constant across ages.

Multiple covariates can be included in a quantile regression model. Table 3.8 shows the results of quantile regression for the first and third quartiles of BMI with (continuous) age, sex, race/ethnicity, and calendar year as covariates. The interpretation is similar to standard regression analysis. For example, the table

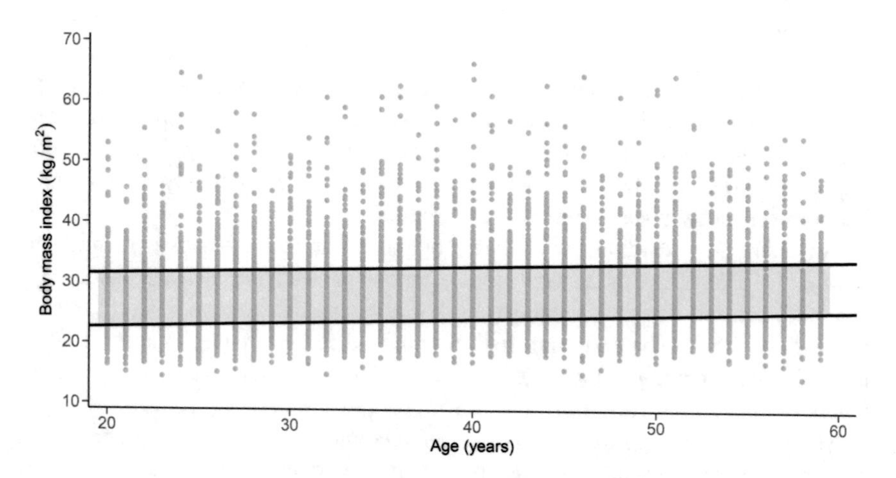

Fig. 3.6 Fitted quantile regression for first and third quartiles of body mass index by age for persons 20–59 years in NHANES sample data for 1999–2000 and 2015–2016

Table 3.8 Quantile regression for the first (1st) and third (3rd) quartiles of body mass index by age for persons age 20–59 years in NHANES sample data for 1999–2000 and 2015–2016

Variable	Coef. (1st)	SE (1st)	*P* (1st)	Coef. (3rd)	SE (3rd)	*P* (3rd)
Intercept	20.29	0.30	<0.001	27.92	0.54	<0.001
SEX = Female	−0.46	0.16	0.003	2.16	0.27	<0.001
RACE = Non-Hispanic black	0.75	0.25	0.003	2.80	0.40	<0.001
RACE = Mexican American	1.83	0.20	<0.001	1.05	0.35	0.003
RACE = Other Hispanic	1.29	0.33	<0.001	0.67	0.45	0.14
RACE = Other/mixed	−1.79	0.22	<0.001	−2.83	0.43	<0.001
AGE	0.08	0.01	<0.001	0.05	0.01	<0.001
YEAR = 2015–2016	0.89	0.16	<0.001	1.85	0.28	<0.001

suggests that the first quartile of BMI increases by 0.08 for each year of age and the third quartile by 0.05. The change with calendar year is noticeably larger for the third quartile (1.85) compared to the first quartile (0.89), which is consistent with BMI skewing higher over time.

3.11 Non-parametric Regression

Section 3.10 considered summaries of the distribution of the outcome besides the mean. Another way that linear regression can be extended beyond the classical setting is to accommodate more flexible forms of the association between covariates and outcomes. One way to do this while still preserving the linear model is to include polynomial and interaction terms. A different way is to use smoothing techniques, also known as *non-parametric regression*.

A linear regression model implies that a one-unit change in any of the covariates is associated with a constant change in the mean of the outcome, regardless of the actual value of the covariate. When there is a more or less constant trend in the outcome as the covariate increases or decreases, this model provides a simple summary of the underlying relationship. For a continuous covariate spanning a wide range of values, however, this assumption can be highly restrictive; it may be more reasonable to assume that the mean of the outcome Y changes slowly and smoothly, but not necessarily linearly, with the covariate X.

An alternative to imposing linearity or indeed any mathematical formula for how $E(Y)$ changes with X would be to model the outcome at each value of X (i.e., for each sub-population defined by X) following the reasoning that close sub-populations (in X) share similar distributions and means of the outcome Y. This is the idea motivating smoothing methods and is a version of a non-parametric regression model.

The simplest way to model this type of relationship between the outcome and a continuous covariate is to divide the covariate into pre-specified groups and to calculate the average within each group. Figure 3.3 showed average BMI levels in

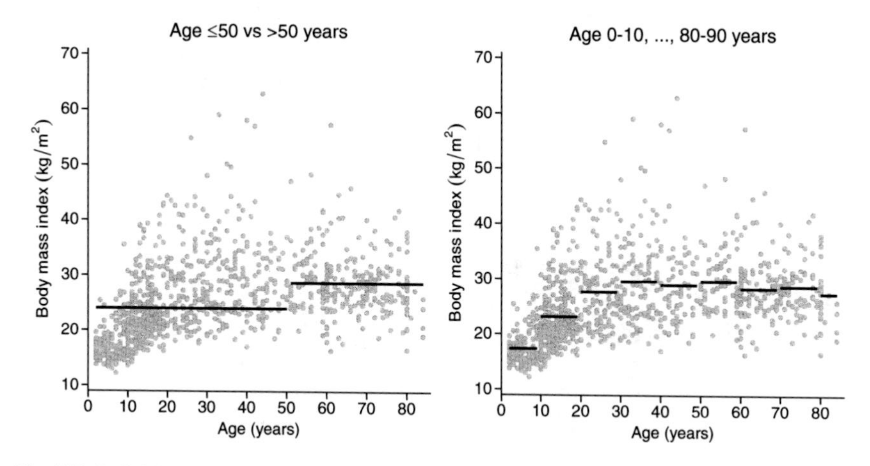

Fig. 3.7 Individual and average body mass index for dichotomized ages and age decades for persons age $\leq$ 85 years in NHANES sample data for 1999–2000 and 2015–2016

groups defined by single ages, but other groupings can be used. Figure 3.7 illustrates this approach using a random sample of 1000 observations from the NHANES sample for all persons age $\leq$ 85 years. The left panel presents the regression line from a dichotomization into two age groups; the right panel presents a more granular breakdown. As more groups are added, the line better reflects the pattern in the data, particularly the non-linearity among the youngest and oldest persons. However, the more granular groupings also result in a smaller sample size in each group and hence a less reliable estimate.

The need to pre-specify the groups and the resulting disconnected lines are obvious drawbacks of the grouping approach. Non-parametric regression predicts the mean of Y for a group with covariate X by borrowing information from neighboring groups. There are many approaches to do this; here we present the simple kernel method that requires minimal mathematical machinery. The uniform kernel method constructs a window of fixed width around each observed X value and predicts the mean of Y at that X value using all the observations in the window. As an example, consider estimating the expected BMI of a person aged 42 years using a uniform kernel with window width 10. This is done by averaging the BMI value of individuals with ages 42 ± 5. Similarly simple averaging is done at each age using the corresponding 10-year window around it. The resulting regression line is shown in Fig. 3.8 along with a semi-transparent rectangle around age 42 and the resulting average (in red).

In uniform kernel regression, all observations in the window contribute equally to the average. Alternatively, we can weight the contribution of each observation according to its distance from the point of interest, decreasing the contribution of further observations. The right panel of Figure 3.8 shows a normal kernel with bandwidth $\sigma = 3$, where the weight of each observation is calculated using a normal density with this standard deviation. For example, the average at age 42

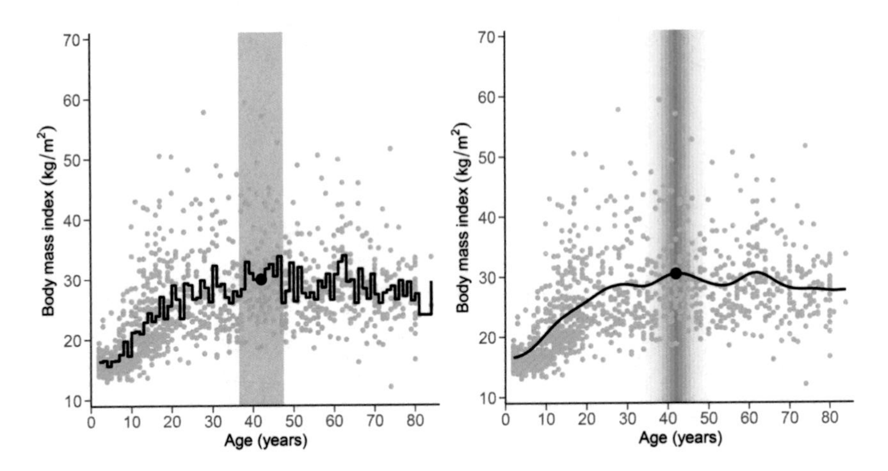

Fig. 3.8 Uniform and normal kernel regression lines for body mass index by age for persons with age $\leq$ 84 years in NHANES sample data for 1999–2000 and 2015–2016. Kernel windows (red semi-transparent vertical strips) for estimating BMI are shown for age 42 years (red dots)

used a weight 0.133 for persons age 42, 0.126 for persons age 41 or 43, 0.106 for persons age 40 or 44, and so on. The semi-transparent rectangles show the diminishing weight applied to observations that are further away from the point of interest (again, age 42 years).

The kernel method provides a graphical estimate of the relationship between the covariate and the outcome. In the current example, BMI increases until adulthood and then flattens. This is an interesting observation, but the contribution of other covariates, such as sex, race/ethnicity, and calendar year, may change the picture. A major limitation of smoothing methods like the kernel approach is that they become difficult to apply when the number of covariates increases. This is sometime referred to as the *curse of dimensionality*, and it occurs because when the covariate space becomes high dimensional, the number of observations within any neighborhood becomes small. Smoothing methods for individual covariates are often used in exploratory analysis, but they should not be used to actually select the covariates to include in regression models or their functional form.

Kernel smoothing is just one approach used for non-parametric regression; another approach uses splines, which are polynomial functions that are combined to fit the observed data. A spline-based approach that assumes additivity but relaxes the linearity assumption is known as a *generalized additive model* [10].

As a final note, our presentation of regression analyses that go beyond classical linear regression only scratches the surface. These techniques can address the objectives defined in Sect. 3.3, but implementing them in practice requires further understanding of their assumptions, interpretation, and, ultimately, their limitations.

3.12 Software and Data

R code to download data and to carry out the examples in this chapter is available at the GitHub page https://roman-gulati.github.io/statistics-for-health-data-science/. In addition to the R packages cited in Chap. 1, this chapter also used the `quantreg` package [11]. The R package `nhanesA` [12] is a utility for downloading NHANES datasets into R.

References

1. Gaskin, D.J., Richard, P.: The economic costs of pain in the United States. J. Pain **13**(8), 715–724 (2012)
2. Centers for Disease Control and Prevention: National health and nutrition examination survey (2020). https://www.cdc.gov/nchs/nhanes/index.htm. Accessed Feb. 12 2020
3. Centers for Disease Control and Prevention: Prevalence of obesity and severe obesity among adults: United States, 2017–2018 (2020). https://www.cdc.gov/nchs/products/databriefs/db360.htm. Accessed July 19 2020
4. Lumley, T., Diehr, P., Emerson, S., Chen, L.: The importance of the normality assumption in large public health data sets. Annu. Rev. Public Health **23**(1), 151–169 (2002)
5. Buse, A.: The likelihood ratio, Wald, and Lagrange multiplier tests: an expository note. Am. Statist. **36**(3), 153–157 (1982)
6. Gelman, A., Hill, J.: Data Analysis Using Regression and Multilevel/Hierarchical Models. Cambridge University Press, Cambridge (2006)
7. Wasserman, L., Roeder, K.: High-dimensional variable selection. Ann. Statist. **37**, 2178–2201 (2009)
8. Taylor, J., Tibshirani, R.J.: Statistical learning and selective inference. Proc. Natl. Acad. Sci. **112**, 7629–7634 (2015)
9. Hong, L., Kuffner, T.A., Martin, R.: On overfitting and post-selection uncertainty assessments. Biometrika **105**, 221–224 (2018)
10. Hastie, T.J., Tibshirani, R.J.: Generalized Additive Models. Monographs on Statistics and Applied Probability, vol. 43. Chapman & Hall/CRC, Boca Raton (1990)
11. Koenker, R.: quantreg: quantile regression (2019). https://CRAN.R-project.org/package=quantreg. R package version 5.52
12. Endres, C.J.: nhanesA: NHANES data retrieval (2018). https://cran.r-project.org/web/packages/nhanesA/index.html. R package version 0.6.5

Chapter 4
Binary and Categorical Outcomes

Abstract This chapter builds a regression framework for binary and categorical outcomes, where the goal is to determine how the distribution of the outcome depends on covariates. The most commonly used model for binary outcomes is logistic regression. We show that logistic regression coefficients are directly interpretable as relative odds of a positive outcome corresponding to changes in covariate values and discuss common misinterpretations of these models. For categorical outcomes, we introduce multinomial regression, which produces coefficients that are interpretable as a multi-category version of relative odds. For both outcomes, we introduce marginal effects as a way to estimate effects of covariates on outcome probabilities rather than odds.

4.1 Introduction

Binary and categorical outcomes arise in many health services and health outcome research studies. Examples of binary outcomes include the presence or absence of certain behaviors or conditions, such as smoking, wearing a seatbelt, or having diabetes. Binary outcomes can also reflect the occurrence or nonoccurrence of disease events, such as hospital re-admission after surgery, in-hospital mortality, or cancer progression after primary treatment.

Categorical or multinomial outcomes have more than two choices. For example, body mass index (BMI) can be categorized as underweight, normal weight, overweight, or obese. While categorical outcomes like BMI have a logical order, outcomes like race/ethnicity have no natural ordering.

Unlike continuous outcomes, categorical outcomes do not have a default numerical scale. Consequently, standard statistical summaries such as the mean, median, or variance are not meaningful. Even if the outcome is coded using numbers, these should not be interpreted quantitatively. For example, a survey may ask

Coauthored by E. Ulloa-Pérez
Department of Biostatistics, University of Washington

R. Etzioni et al., *Statistics for Health Data Science*, Springer Texts in Statistics,
https://doi.org/10.1007/978-3-030-59889-1_4

respondents to report their health status by choosing 1 (excellent), 2 (very good), 3 (good), 4 (fair), or 5 (poor). But we cannot simply replace the categories by their numerical codes and analyze them as if they were continuous measurements, as if the difference between 2 (very good) and 3 (good) is the same as the difference between 4 (fair) and 5 (poor). This is even more obvious for categorical outcomes that do not have a natural order, such as race/ethnicity, type of medical insurance, or provider specialty. Even though numbers are frequently used to code binary or categorical outcomes, they do not necessarily represent ordinal measurements.

Due to the discrete nature of binary and categorical outcomes, we cannot use standard linear regression to study relationships with other variables. Therefore, another statistical approach is needed to analyze categorical outcome data. In this chapter, we start with the simpler case of binary outcomes. We introduce the logistic regression model using an indicator of obesity as our outcome, and we compare our analysis to standard linear regression. In Sect. 4.8, we cover regression modeling of general categorical outcomes building on logistic regression for binary outcomes.

4.2 Binary Outcomes

A binary outcome, Y, can take one of two possible values that we can generically label positive or negative and denote as 1 or 0, respectively. For example, in a study of 10-day re-admissions after hospitalization, a patient may be readmitted ($Y = 1$) or not ($Y = 0$); in a study of chronic disease, a patient may have diabetes ($Y = 1$) or not ($Y = 0$); in a study of medical costs in a given year, an individual may have positive ($Y = 1$) or zero ($Y = 0$) medical expenditures.

We can think of a binary outcome as a random variable with distribution comprised of the probabilities that $Y = 1$ and $Y = 0$. (This is called a *Bernoulli* distribution; see Chap. 2.) Because these two probabilities must sum to one, the distribution is completely determined by one of the two probabilities, which is conventionally taken to be the probability of a positive outcome, $P(Y = 1)$. When considering the association between a covariate and a binary outcome, therefore, we need simply to understand how this probability is associated with the covariate.

The convention of replacing the levels of the binary outcome, like "obese" and "not obese," with the numbers 1 and 0 is done for notational convenience. Regardless of the application setting, we can observe that the mean of the binary outcome Y is the same as the proportion of positive outcomes, or $E(Y) = P(Y = 1)$.

In Chap. 3, we discussed linear regression as a method to study how the mean of a continuous outcome changes across sub-populations. For binary outcomes, we will study how the proportion of positive outcomes changes across sub-populations. As a practical example, we will examine how the proportion of obese persons changes over time and by age.

We will use data from the National Health and Nutrition Examination Survey (NHANES), which is the most authoritative source of data on the body mass index (BMI) in the United States. BMI is a measure of body fat based on height and weight and is calculated as the body mass in kilograms divided by the square of the body height in meters. The World Health Organization defines an adult with BMI of 30.0 or higher as obese. There are countless studies of BMI trends in the United States, sounding an alarm about the obesity epidemic and its implications for chronic disease morbidity and mortality. Although the NHANES follows a complex survey design including stratification, clustering, and weighting, these topics are postponed to Chap. 9; we do not use the survey design variables to produce the results in this chapter.

In Chap. 3, we studied the change in mean BMI between 1999–2000 and 2015–2016; in this chapter, we focus on the change in the proportion of obese persons over this interval. As before, we restrict attention to persons age 20–59 years because trends in children and the elderly may be subject to different considerations. Coding the response variable as a binary outcome instead of a continuous outcome addresses a different scientific question, which may have its own implications for population health and public health policy.

4.2.1 *Two-Way Tables*

Our NHANES dataset include 6864 individuals age 20–59 years: 3046 from the 1999–2000 survey and 3818 from the 2015–2016 survey. Mean BMI increased from 28.4 kg/m^2 in 1999–2000 to 29.6 kg/m^2 in 2015–2016, an increase of 1.2 units. This might not be a public health concern if it were due to changes in BMI within the underweight or normal weight groups. However, it would be concerning if it indicated an increase in overweight and obese persons as this would affect the incidence of chronic diseases, such as heart failure and diabetes.

The two-way table shown in Table 4.1 presents the frequency of obese and non-obese persons for the two calendar years. The table shows an increase in the proportion obese from 32.5% to 40.4% in 15 years.

The absolute 8% increase has the same meaning regardless of the baseline proportion in 1999–2000. Sometimes the relative increase is reported, in which case the baseline proportion matters. For example, when the baseline proportion is 5%, a 10% relative increase translates into an absolute 0.5% increase; when the baseline proportion is 50%, a 10% relative increase translates into an absolute 5% increase.

The relative increase is often expressed using a *risk ratio* or *relative risk* (RR). In the obesity example, the RR for obesity in 2015–2016 relative to 1999–2000 is calculated as:

Table 4.1 Frequency of obese and non-obese persons age 20–59 years in NHANES sample data for 1999–2000 and 2015–2016

Year	Not obese	Obese	Total
1999–2000	1899 (67.5%)	914 (32.5%)	2813 (100.0%)
2015–2016	2165 (59.6%)	1469 (40.4%)	3634 (100.0%)

$$\text{RR} = \frac{\text{Proportion obese in 2015–2016}}{\text{Proportion obese in 1999–2000}} = \frac{0.404}{0.325} = 1.24.$$

An RR close to 1 means there is little relative change; an RR that is substantially smaller or larger than 1 means there is a substantial relative change. In this example, the RR of 1.24 means the proportion obese in 2015–2016 represented a 24% increase relative to 1999–2000. The change in RR across values of a covariate (calendar year in this example) measures the strength of association between the outcome and that covariate.

An alternative measure of association is the *odds ratio* or *relative odds* (OR). The "odds" is a well-known quantity in gambling. It is itself a ratio, namely, the probability of the positive outcome divided by the probability of the negative outcome, i.e., $P(Y = 1)/P(Y = 0)$. When the covariate is binary, the OR is simply the ratio of the odds of the outcome in each group. In our obesity example, calendar year is a binary covariate, and the OR is defined as:

$$\text{OR} = \frac{(\text{Proportion obese in 2015–2016})/(\text{Proportion not obese in 2015–2016})}{(\text{Proportion obese in 1999–2000})/(\text{Proportion not obese in 1999–2000})}.$$

Calculation of the OR from the two-way table is simple; it is just the product of the diagonal elements divided by the product of the off-diagonal elements:

$$\begin{aligned} \text{OR} &= \frac{(\text{Number not obese in 1999–2000}) \times (\text{Number obese in 2015–2016})}{(\text{Number obese in 1999–2000}) \times (\text{Number not obese in 2015–2016})} \\ &= \frac{1899 \times 1469}{914 \times 2165} = 1.41. \end{aligned}$$

The OR is symmetric, with the roles of the outcome and the covariate interchangeable. This is a desirable property for a general measure of association; the correlation coefficient for continuous data is another example of a symmetric measure of association.

While the RR is intuitive and readily interpretable, the OR is neither. However, as we will see, the OR is what is typically modeled. Consequently, it is helpful to observe a few properties of the OR:

1. The OR indicates the same direction of association as the RR. If there is no association between the outcome and covariate, both the OR and RR equal 1. Also, the OR > 1 whenever the RR > 1, and the OR < 1 whenever the RR < 1.
2. If the outcome is associated with the covariate, the OR is always farther from 1 than the RR. For example, if OR $= 1.41$, we know that $1 <$ RR < 1.41.
3. For rare positive outcomes, the OR and the RR are similar. Since odds $= P(Y = 1)/P(Y = 0)$ is close to $P(Y = 1)$ when $P(Y = 0)$ is close to 1, the ratio of odds is close to the ratio of probabilities.

The third property is handy because it means we can interpret the OR as being approximately equal to the RR when positive outcomes are uncommon. Unfortunately, this is not true when positive outcomes are common. When $P(Y =$

Table 4.2 Risk ratio (RR) and odds ratio (OR) for selected probabilities of positive outcomes

$P(Y = 1 \mid X = 0)$	$P(Y = 1 \mid X = 1)$	RR	OR
0.01	0.02	2.00	2.02
0.01	0.04	4.00	4.12
0.05	0.10	2.00	2.11
0.05	0.20	4.00	4.75
0.10	0.20	2.00	2.25
0.10	0.40	4.00	6.00

1) is non-trivial, $P(Y = 0)$ is not close to 1, and this can make the OR and RR dissimilar. Table 4.2 shows the RR and the OR for different instances of a setting with a binary covariate X. When the probabilities of a positive outcome are very small, the OR is close to the RR. But when the probabilities of positive outcomes are not very small, the OR is not close to the RR.

4.3 Linear Regression with a Binary Outcome

Can we use a linear regression to examine the association between a binary outcome and a covariate? Figure 4.1 shows a scatterplot of obesity status versus age in the NHANES sample data. To avoid "overplotting" points with the same age and obesity status, the size of each point is proportional to the number of observations. While a linear regression line can technically be calculated, it is not immediately clear what it represents.

Thinking of each age as defining a sub-population, we can try to model the proportion of obese persons across sub-populations. Noting that the proportion of obese persons at each age is just the mean of the obesity outcome at that age, this framing of the problem exactly mirrors the idea behind linear regression. The dots in Fig. 4.2 show the proportion of obese persons at each age. The fitted linear regression is shown as the blue line.

While the linear model reasonably captures the proportion of obese persons across the age range considered in this example, the linear regression formulation does not constrain the predicted probabilities to be between zero and one. When outcomes are rare, the predictions may even be outside these bounds. We would not trust a model that could predict the percent of obese persons to be -12% or 131%! Furthermore, we should be concerned about making any inferences when a linear regression that assumes a continuous, normally distributed outcome variable is applied to a discrete, non-normal outcome.

Binary regression constrains the regression equation to be between zero and one, and it represents a coherent way of addressing the discrete, non-normal nature of the data. The orange line in Fig. 4.2 shows the prediction from a logistic regression, the most popular type of binary regression. In our obesity example, the logistic regression is very close to the linear model for the range of data considered, but this is not always the case.

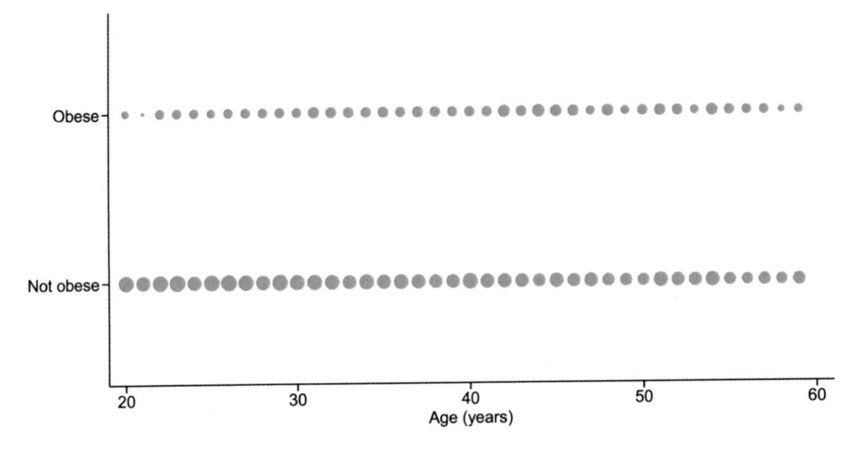

Fig. 4.1 Scatterplot of obesity status versus age for persons age 20–59 years in NHANES sample data for 1999–2000 and 2015–2016. Dot size is proportional to number of observations

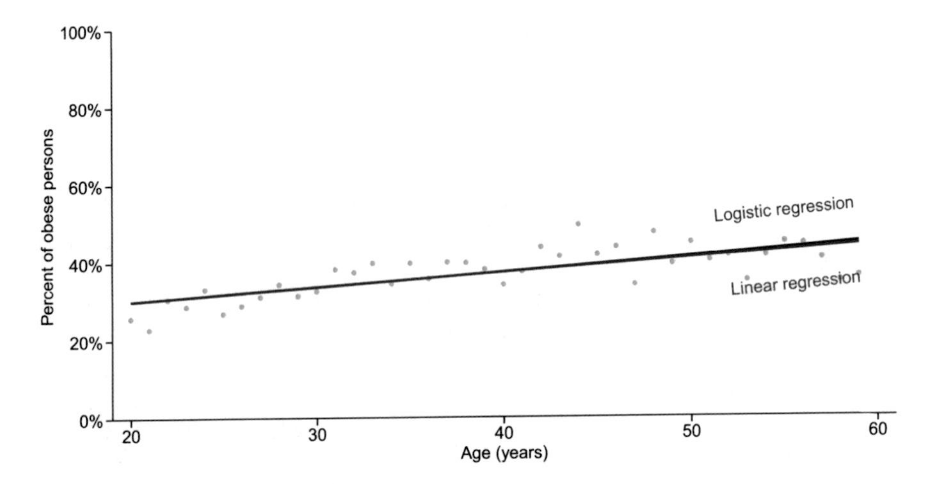

Fig. 4.2 Percent of obese persons age 20–59 years in NHANES sample data for 1999–2000 and 2015–2016 with linear and logistic regression lines

4.4 Logistic Regression

Logistic regression is a way to model the association between the probability of a positive outcome $P(Y = 1)$ and one or more covariates X so that the regression line stays within the interval [0, 1]. How is this done? To understand the reasoning behind logistic regression, recall that linear regression of a continuous outcome Y on a set of covariates $X_1, \ldots, X_k$ has two parts:

$$Y = \beta_0 + \beta_1 X_1 + \cdots + \beta_k X_k + \epsilon,$$

where $\beta_0 + \beta_1 X_1 + \cdots + \beta_k X_k$ is the systematic part, determining the mean of Y in the sub-populations defined by the Xs, and ϵ is the error term that reflects random deviation of a subject from the mean in that sub-population. However, with a binary outcome, this approach fails because (1) the systematic part for the probability $P(Y = 1)$ can be smaller than 0 or larger than 1, an undesirable possibility, and (2) the error term has a very limited range of possible values and depends on the systematic part since the sum of the two parts must be either 0 or 1.

As the formulation "outcome = systematic part + error part" fails, we must adopt a different formulation to model binary outcomes. A natural way is to think about the outcome of each person as being a result of a binary experiment, such as tossing a coin. The systematic part defines the probability of "success" of the experiment, corresponding to $P(Y = 1)$, and the random part of the model is replaced by a random result of the experiment. Since the linear formulation for the systematic part does not guarantee that the model will conform to the [0, 1] range, a mathematical "trick" is required. This mathematical trick is simply a transformation of the systematic part from the linear formulation. The most commonly used transformation is the logistic function, which yields:

$$P(Y_i = 1) = \frac{\exp(\beta_0 + \beta_1 X_{1i} + \cdots + \beta_k X_{ki})}{1 + \exp(\beta_0 + \beta_1 X_{1i} + \cdots + \beta_k X_{ki})}, \tag{4.1}$$

where Y_i is the outcome of subject i and $X_{1i}, \ldots, X_{ki}$ are the covariates. Let's think about why this model works. Suppose that we have only one continuous covariate, X_1, and suppose also that β_1 is positive. Then when X_1 is positive and increases in magnitude, both the numerator and the denominator in Eq. (4.1) increase, and their ratio approaches 1. Conversely, when X_1 is negative and increases in magnitude, the numerator approaches 0, and the denominator approaches 1, so the ratio in Eq. (4.1) approaches 0. More generally, the numerator is always less than the denominator by construction, so the ratio is always between 0 and 1. Thus, this function is a perfect candidate to satisfy the requirements of a regression model for probabilities.

In Eq. (4.1), the effect of the Xs is additive and linear before the transformation, but the transformation generates a complicated, non-linear function for $P(Y = 1)$. An equivalent formulation of this model preserves the linear specification for the Xs but applies the inverse transformation to Y. This transformation is called the *logit*, and the formulation is as follows:

$$\text{logit}[P(Y_i = 1)] = \log\left[\frac{P(Y_i = 1)}{P(Y_i = 0)}\right] = \beta_0 + \beta_1 X_{1i} + \cdots + \beta_k X_{ki}. \tag{4.2}$$

Note that the logit is simply the natural logarithm of the odds. Thus, the logistic regression model assumes that the log of the odds depends linearly on the covariates.

The transformation that produces logistic regression is only one of several available for binary outcomes. In general, to convert the range of the systematic part to be between 0 and 1, any function that converts a number in the range $(-\infty, +\infty)$ to a number in [0, 1] in a sensible way will do the trick. Thinking back to the statistical background in Chap. 2, we're familiar with several such transformations because the *cumulative distribution function* (CDF) of a statistical distribution converts a random variable from its original range to the range [0, 1]. Recall the CDF of a random variable Y at value y represents the probability that Y is less than or equal to y, a probability that increases from 0 at the lowest extreme of Y to 1 at the highest extreme of Y. Therefore, the CDF for any random variable defined over the range $(-\infty, +\infty)$ could serve as a candidate transformation. The probit model, well-known in econometrics and finance, uses the CDF of a standard normal random variable to transform the systematic part. The logistic model in Eq. (4.1) does the same thing, in fact, with the CDF of a logistic random variable.

The most obvious consequence of the logistic (or any CDF-based) transformation is that we have converted a linear model into a non-linear one. The left-hand side of the regression equation is still the mean or expectation of Y, $E(Y)$, since $E(Y) = P(Y = 1)$, but the right-hand side is no longer simply a linear combination of the Xs. We can rewrite the model, as in Eq. (4.2), so that the right-hand side is linear. However, the left-hand side is then not the mean of the outcome but rather a more complicated function of the outcome. The popularity of the logistic transformation stems from the fact that this transformation is statistically meaningful, so the results are interpretable in terms of odds and odds ratios. As we shall show, however, this is still subject to frequent misinterpretation.

4.5 Interpretation of a Logistic Regression

4.5.1 A Single Binary Covariate

Due to the form of the transformed response variable, logistic regression tells us how the log odds of a positive outcome ($Y = 1$) changes when one of the Xs change. To illustrate how we interpret a logistic regression, let's repeat the analysis in Sect. 4.2 where Y is the indicator of obesity and X is a single binary covariate taking the value 0 for year 1999–2000 and the value 1 for year 2015–2016. The results of this model are summarized in Table 4.3.

Table 4.3 Logistic regression of obese persons age 20–59 years in NHANES sample data for 1999–2000 and 2015–2016

Predictor	Coefficient	SE	P-value
Intercept	−0.731	0.040	<0.001
YEAR = 2015–2016	0.343	0.053	<0.001

Table 4.3 is similar to that obtained in linear regression, where the standard error (SE) is a measure of uncertainty of the coefficient estimate and a p-value is given for the hypothesis test that each coefficient is equal to 0. As in the linear model, the p-value is calculated by dividing the coefficient by its standard error and comparing the result to a standard normal distribution.

How can we interpret the estimate of 0.343 for the association with year? This is not interpreted as the expected increase in Y on the original scale; it must be interpreted on the log odds scale. Symbolically we have:

$$\text{logit}[P(Y = 1 \mid X = 1)] - \text{logit}[P(Y = 1 \mid X = 0)] = 0.343.$$

If we exponentiate both sides, we get:

$$\text{odds}[P(Y = 1 \mid X = 1)]/\text{odds}[P(Y = 1 \mid X = 0)] = \exp(0.343) = 1.41.$$

The exponentiated log odds ratio is simply the odds ratio. Because the response variable was log transformed, the logistic model induces a multiplicative effect on the odds of $Y = 1$. Thus, while linear regression is an additive model for the mean of the outcome, logistic regression is a multiplicative model for the odds.

Also notice that the result in this example (OR $=$ 1.41) is exactly the result we obtained in Sect. 4.2 using the two-way table. Now look at the corresponding probabilities; this can be done with the help of Eq. (4.1):

$$P(Y = 1 \mid X = 0) = \frac{\exp(-0.731)}{1 + \exp(-0.731)} = 0.325$$

$$P(Y = 1 \mid X = 1) = \frac{\exp(-0.731 + 0.343)}{1 + \exp(-0.731 + 0.343)} = 0.404.$$

Again, these are exactly the numbers obtained using the two-way table in Sect. 4.2. This is not a coincidence. A logistic regression with a single binary covariate is quite simple: it just replicates the calculations of the proportions and their odds in the comparison of two groups.

4.5.2 *The General Case*

In this subsection, we consider models with multiple covariates and work through issues with interpreting the results of a logistic regression. We fit a logistic regression to the indicator of obesity (OBESE) with binary covariates SEX (with reference level male) and YEAR (with reference level 1999–2000), a five-level categorical covariate RACE (with reference level non-Hispanic white) coded as a set of four dummy variables and continuous covariate AGE (centered at 20 years, the youngest age in our analysis). For this setup, the reference group is the sub-population of non-Hispanic white men age 20 in 1999–2000.

Table 4.4 provides the fraction obese corresponding to each level of each covariate. For non-reference levels, the odds of being obese relative to the reference level is also shown. The OR for SEX is greater than 1, suggesting the risk of being obese is higher for women than for men. This can also be seen by comparing the percentages: about 32% of men are obese compared to 41% of women. For RACE, we see that the OR of the Other/mixed group is smaller than 1, indicating that persons in this group tend to be less at risk of obesity than the reference group (non-Hispanic white persons). The ORs for the other RACE groups are greater than 1, and their order matches the ordering of the percentages of obese persons.

Table 4.5 provides the results of a logistic regression with multiple covariates. The baseline category for YEAR is 1999–2000; the coefficient estimate for YEAR = 2015–2016 is 0.44. This tells us that, given AGE, SEX, and RACE, persons in 2015–2016 have a 0.44 increased log odds of being obese compared with persons in 1999–2000. The corresponding odds ratio is 1.55; thus, in 2015–2016, the odds of being obese are 1.55 times higher than in 1999–2000. The ORs for the multivariate regression have a conditional interpretation in that they are interpretable

Table 4.4 Univariate summaries of selected categorical variables for obese persons age 20–59 years in NHANES sample data in 1999–2000 and 2015–2016

Variable	Sample, *n*	Obese, *n* (%)	Odds ratio
SEX = Male	2972	954 (32.1%)	Reference
SEX = Female	3475	1429 (41.1%)	1.48
RACE = Non-Hispanic white	2228	732 (32.9%)	Reference
RACE = Non-Hispanic black	1364	615 (45.1%)	1.68
RACE = Mexican American	1428	589 (41.2%)	1.43
RACE = Other Hispanic	663	271 (40.9%)	1.41
RACE = Other/mixed	764	176 (23.0%)	0.61
YEAR = 1999–2000	2813	914 (32.5%)	Reference
YEAR = 2015–2016	3634	1469 (40.4%)	1.41

Table 4.5 Multivariate logistic regression of being obese for persons age 20–59 years in NHANES sample data in 1999–2000 and 2015–2016 showing each estimated coefficient ($\hat{\beta}$), standard error (SE), P-value for the hypothesis of no association ($\hat{\beta} = 0$), odds ratio (OR = $\exp(\hat{\beta})$), and 95% confidence interval (CI) for the OR ($\exp(\hat{\beta} \pm 1.96 \times \text{SE})$)

Predictor	Coefficient	SE	P-value	OR	95% CI
Intercept	−1.46	0.08	<0.001		
SEX = Female	0.40	0.05	<0.001	1.48	(1.34,1.65)
RACE = Non-Hispanic black	0.47	0.07	<0.001	1.60	(1.39,1.84)
RACE = Mexican American	0.39	0.07	<0.001	1.48	(1.28,1.70)
RACE = Other Hispanic	0.24	0.09	<0.01	1.27	(1.06,1.53)
RACE = Other/mixed	−0.64	0.10	<0.001	0.53	(0.43,0.64)
AGE	0.02	0.00	<0.001	1.02	(1.01,1.02)
YEAR = 2015–2016	0.44	0.06	<0.001	1.55	(1.39,1.72)

as the change in the odds of being obese for the sub-population defined by the values of all the other covariates.

The interpretation of the coefficient in a logistic regression is similar in principle to a linear regression setting: we can think of it as the estimated effect of a one-unit change in the covariate holding the other covariates fixed. (Note: we use the term "effect" here for conciseness and not to imply causality [1].) However, in a logistic regression, we are not estimating the effect on $E(Y)$—we're estimating the effect on the log odds of $Y = 1$. Thus, the coefficient of a categorical covariate is the estimated difference in log odds compared to the reference level. For example, being a woman is associated with a 0.40 difference in the log odds of being obese compared to being a man. Alternatively, being a woman is associated with 1.48 times the odds of being obese compared to being a man. The estimated association between covariate and log odd or odds of the outcome is the same for any race, persons of any age, and in either survey calendar year.

In the case of a continuous covariate, interpretation is similar. For example, being 1 year older is associated with an increase in the log odds of being obese of 0.02 or, alternatively, an OR of 1.02. This estimated association does not depend on the specific value of age, and it does not depend on the specific values of the other covariates. To estimate the effect of a 10-year increase in age, we simply multiply the coefficient by 10, obtaining a difference in log odds of 0.2 and a corresponding OR of $\exp(0.2) = 1.22$.

So far we have discussed how changes in covariates are associated with the log odds or odds of a positive response. But we often want to know how changes in covariates are associated with the *probability* of a positive response. This is generally easier to understand. As noted above (Sect. 4.2.1), the OR is sometimes interpretable as an approximate relative risk—i.e., a ratio of probabilities rather than a ratio of odds—but this interpretation is only valid when the outcome is rare.

When positive outcomes are not rare, the OR can be quite different from the relative risk. For example, a 1999 article in *The New England Journal of Medicine* that compared rates of referral to cardiac catheterization in African American and white patients found an OR of 0.6 [2]. This result was considered to be evidence of a dramatic racial disparity in the receipt of cardiac catheterization, but the corresponding risk ratio was actually 0.93 [3]—much closer to 1! The two measures were so different owing to a relatively high fraction of each group receiving a referral (92% of white patients and 89% of black patients). This left rather small denominators for the odds in each group, which led to an odds ratio that completely misrepresented the relatively minor difference between the probabilities. It is not infrequent to see results of logistic regression analyses interpreted in this way—the natural language of risk is probability, not odds. So, what if we really want to understand our logistic regression results in terms of relative probabilities or differences in probabilities instead of relative odds and differences in log odds? This is the topic of the next section.

4.6 Interpretation on the Probability Scale

4.6.1 Estimating Probabilities

Equation (4.1) tells us how to calculate the probability of a positive outcome for any sub-population. For example, the probability of a positive outcome in the reference group of non-Hispanic white (NHW) men age 20 years in 1999–2000 is:

$$P(Y = 1 \mid \text{NHW, Male, 20}) = \frac{\exp(-1.46)}{1 + \exp(-1.46)} = 0.188.$$

If we want to estimate the probability for an otherwise similar woman, we simply add the coefficient of SEX:

$$P(Y = 1 \mid \text{NHW, Female, 20}) = \frac{\exp(-1.46 + 0.40)}{1 + \exp(-1.46 + 0.40)} = 0.257,$$

and if we want to estimate the probability for an otherwise similar woman age 52 years, we simply add the coefficient of AGE times 32 ($= 52 - 20$):

$$P(Y = 1 \mid \text{NHW, Female, 52}) = \frac{\exp(-1.46 + 0.40 + 0.02 \times 32)}{1 + \exp(-1.46 + 0.40 + 0.02 \times 32)} = 0.397.$$

Because interpreting ORs is not straightforward, we would like to define the effect of a covariate on the probability of a positive outcome, $P(Y = 1)$. There are two types of effects for a covariate X:

1. An *additive effect* (AE), equal to the absolute change in $P(Y = 1 \mid X)$ for a one-unit change in X:

$$\text{AE} = P(Y = 1 \mid X = 1) - P(Y = 1 \mid X = 0).$$

2. A *multiplicative effect* (ME) equal to the relative change in $P(Y = 1 \mid X)$ for a one-unit change in X:

$$\text{ME} = P(Y = 1 \mid X = 1)/P(Y = 1 \mid X = 0).$$

The additive effect is sometimes referred to as a *risk difference*. The multiplicative effect is the previously defined risk ratio. For either effect, we would ideally like an estimate that does not depend on the specific values of the other covariates, just as in linear regression.

Figure 4.3 shows why this is a tall order. The figure shows predicted probabilities of being obese implied by the fitted logistic regression in Table 4.5 for persons in race category Other/mixed and different values of AGE, SEX, and YEAR. One can observe that the predicted probabilities are not quite linear in the covariates. This

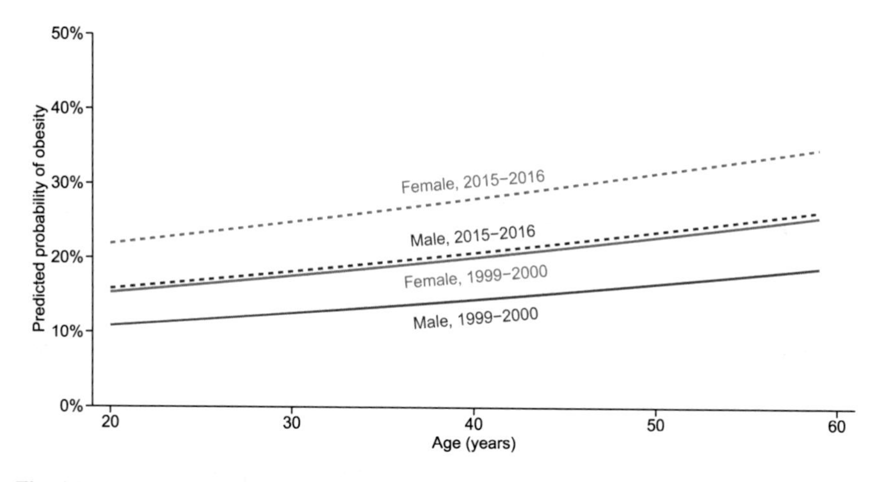

Fig. 4.3 Predicted probabilities of being obese for persons age 20–59 years in race category Other/mixed in NHANES sample data for 1999–2000 and 2015–2016

is a consequence of the logit transformation that converted the model from a linear to a non-linear model. The model is only linear on the log odds scale—not on the original probability scale.

In fact, not only do the predicted probabilities increase non-linearly with age, but the effect of year differs depending on age. This is reminiscent of the normal linear model with an interaction between age and year, which was a non-linear model. The regression equation in this case does not explicitly include an interaction, but when converted to the probability scale, it is also non-linear.

The top panel of Fig. 4.4 shows the difference between the predicted probabilities in years 2015–2016 and 1999–2000 across values of SEX and AGE for RACE = Other/mixed. If the model were additive and linear on the probability scale, the differences would be similar for men and women and constant across ages. However, this is not the case. In fact, the additive effect of YEAR depends on AGE and SEX; the absolute change in BMI over time is greater for older people and for women. We refer to this effect as a *conditional additive effect*—the additive effect depends on the exact values of the other covariates: AGE, SEX, and RACE. The *conditional multiplicative effect* is defined similarly as the conditional ratio of the probabilities of being obese in the later and earlier years. The middle panel of Fig. 4.4 shows this ratio across values of SEX and AGE for RACE = Other/mixed. In contrast to the absolute change, the relative change over time in BMI is lower for older persons and for women.

In Fig. 4.4, only the odds ratio (bottom panel) is the same across ages and for men and women. In logistic regression, the odds ratio is the single measure of association that does not depend on the specific values of other covariates. The question that remains, then, is whether we can estimate an additive or multiplicative effect on the probability scale (i.e., "risk differences").

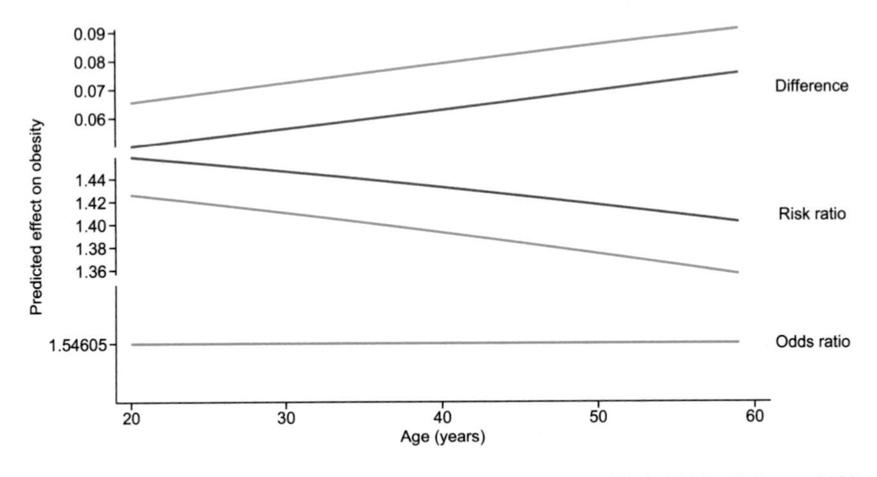

Fig. 4.4 Difference, risk ratio, and odds ratio for being obese in 2015–2016 relative to 1999–2000 based on predicted probabilities for men (blue) and women (green) age 20–59 years in race category Other/mixed in NHANES sample data

4.6.2 Marginal Effects

One way to estimate the effect of a covariate on the probability scale is to convert the *conditional* additive or multiplicative effect to a *marginal* effect (see Chap. 2 for discussion of conditional versus marginal means). Here, we are using the term "marginal" in its technical sense, meaning as an average. In Chap. 2, we learned that we could obtain a marginal quantity by appropriately averaging the corresponding conditional quantities.

In the logistic regression setting, the marginal additive effect of YEAR is an average of the conditional additive effects, defined above, over the distribution of all the other covariates: AGE, SEX, and RACE. The result is meaningful as a difference in the probability of being obese in 2015–2016 versus 1999–2000; it is adjusted for all covariates, and it does not depend on their specific values since it averages over them.

Estimation of a marginal effect consists of a two-step process:

(1) Estimate the conditional effect of interest (e.g., of YEAR) based on the observed data.
(2) Average the estimates in (1) over the joint distribution of all other covariates.

To estimate the marginal effect of YEAR in the obesity example, step (2) averages the conditional effect estimates over the distributions of AGE, SEX, and RACE. This may make sense theoretically, but how can we implement it practically in our sample?

The *recycled prediction* method [4] implements step (2) by averaging over the empirical distribution of the other covariates (i.e., the set of values actually observed in the data), yielding a sample average version of step (2). We explain how the method works using the association between BMI and YEAR as an illustrative example.

(1) For each person in the data, calculate a person-specific conditional additive effect as the difference between their predicted probabilities:

$$\widehat{P}(Y = 1 \mid \text{YEAR} = 2015\text{–}2016) - \widehat{P}(Y = 1 \mid \text{YEAR} = 1999\text{–}2000).$$

The first predicted probability is calculated from the fitted logistic regression by setting YEAR to 1 (2015–2016), and the second is calculated by setting YEAR to 0 (1999–2000) *fixing the other covariates at the values observed for that person*. Thus, two predicted probabilities are calculated for each person. The differences are individual-level conditional effects and are presented in the top panel of Fig. 4.4 for persons in the race category Other/mixed.

(2) Calculate the sample average of the individual-level conditional effects. This is the same thing as calculating a weighted average of the conditional effects over the empirical (sample) distribution of the other covariates. This produces a sample average version of step (2) above.

Variance estimation for the marginal additive effect is generally performed using a technique called the delta method or by numerical methods such as bootstrapping (Chap. 7); the package `margins` in R [5] can do all the necessary calculations. The variance can be used to construct a confidence interval for the marginal additive effect.

The marginal additive effect for YEAR is estimated as 0.102 with 95% confidence interval $(0.077, 0.128)$. Thus, the fraction of adults that are obese in 2015–2016 is about 10% higher than in 1999–2000. Even though this estimate averages over the other covariates and therefore does not explicitly depend on them, it does depend on their distribution in the sample. If the sample distribution of the other covariates is not representative of the population distribution, the result may not generalize to the population. Finally, although recycled predictions may be reported using terms like "effects" and so may seem to suggest a causal framework, this is simply convenient nomenclature, and results should not be interpreted causally unless causal inference methods are employed (Chap. 8).

As a check on our estimate of the marginal additive effect, we can compare it with the estimated coefficient of YEAR from a linear regression model of BMI on YEAR. In fact, the estimated coefficient from linear regression may be thought of as a conditional additive effect on the probability scale that does not depend on the specific values of the other covariates. Because it is independent of the specific values of the other covariates, averaging over their distribution will yield the same estimate. It is therefore both a conditional and a marginal additive effect. The coefficient estimate from a linear regression should approximate the marginal additive effect from the logistic regression, although the estimated standard errors will likely differ. Applying a linear regression model gives an effect of 0.098 for YEAR with a 95% confidence interval $(0.074, 0.123)$, which is very similar to our marginal additive effect in this example.

If interest instead focuses on multiplicative effects, we can calculate the ratio:

$$\frac{P(Y = 1 \mid \text{YEAR} = 2015\text{–}2016)}{P(Y = 1 \mid \text{YEAR} = 1999\text{–}2000)}$$

rather than the difference in step (1) and average over all the estimates. This will yield an average risk ratio over the sample. Estimating variance, however, can be more complicated; for more information on this topic, see, for instance, Zou [6]. Alternatively, bootstrapping, discussed in Chap. 7, can be employed.

4.7 Model Building and Assessment

The principles of building a logistic regression model and assessing its fit are similar to those used for linear regression models (Chap. 3), but certain additional considerations apply due to the binary nature of the response variable. As in linear regression, the objective of the analysis is paramount. If the goal of the analysis is to conduct inference to test a pre-specified hypothesis, then model adequacy will hinge on whether the model accurately reflects the data-generating mechanism. If the goal of the analysis is to deliver a conclusion that points to a causal relationship, then model adequacy will rest on whether the model properly accounts for other potential confounding variables. And if the goal is to predict the occurrence of an event or of a condition encoded using a binary response, then predictive accuracy will be key. In this section, we review some of the commonly used tools for assessing model adequacy and comparing models for binary outcomes.

4.7.1 Model Comparison: AIC and BIC

The parameters of logistic regression are estimated by maximum likelihood, where the parameters $\beta_0, \beta_1, \ldots, \beta_k$ in Eq. (4.1) are chosen to maximize the likelihood of obtaining the data observed. We can test for the adequacy of a model with fewer covariates, say a model that assumes there is no effect of the race variable in the obesity example, by omitting those variables, re-estimating the regression model, and comparing the likelihood of the observed data with and without those variables. This is the *likelihood ratio test* for nested models, described in Chap. 3.

In Chap. 3, we also introduced the *Akaike Information Criterion* (AIC) and *Bayesian Information Criterion* (BIC) for comparison of nested and non-nested models. These are versions of the maximized log-likelihood L of a model M that include an added penalty for model complexity. These statistics provide a metric for model selection in which added complexity is only worthwhile if it pays for itself by adequately improving the likelihood. The goal is to find the model that minimizes the AIC (or BIC). The two statistics are similar, but the BIC invokes a more severe penalty for model complexity that also depends on the sample size n, so it may select simpler, more parsimonious models than the AIC in certain cases. Chapter 3 provides more detailed discussion of these model comparison metrics. Here we reiterate that the models being compared need to preserve the response variable (e.g., one cannot compare a linear regression to a logistic regression) and need to pertain to the same set of observations.

4.7.2 Model Calibration: Hosmer–Lemeshow Test

The maximum likelihood estimates of the parameters have several appealing properties. For example, the sum of predicted probabilities of being obese (i.e., the sum of predicted $P(Y = 1 \mid X)$ over the sample) exactly equals the observed number of obese persons. Moreover, this is true not only for the total number of obese persons in the sample but also within each discrete sub-population defined by SEX, RACE, or YEAR. Thus, the predicted number of obese persons in 1999–2000 equals the observed number of obese persons in that survey year. In other words, the model is perfectly calibrated when looking at each level of a binary or categorical variable.

But what about sub-populations defined by continuous variables or by more than one discrete variable? We say that a model is well calibrated if the number of obese persons it predicts in each possible sub-population is close to the observed number in that group. For example, we would like the predicted number of obese non-Hispanic white men in the age group 30–35 in 1999–2000 to closely match the observed number in that group. Since there are many possible sub-populations of this kind to look at, a systematic way to assess model calibration is needed. A now common approach was suggested by Hosmer and Lemeshow in their highly cited paper [7].

The Hosmer-Lemeshow approach compares observed and predicted quantities as follows:

1. Order the observations according to their predicted $P(Y = 1 \mid X)$, so the person with the lowest predicted probability of being obese is first, and the person with the highest predicted probability of being obese is last.
2. Partition the ordered observations into m equal-sized groups. For example, if $m = 10$, partition the ordered observations into ten groups, with each group comprising approximately 10% of the sample. The first group contains observations with the lowest predicted probabilities, and the last group contains those observations with the highest predicted probabilities.
3. Create a two-way contingency table by cross-tabulating counts of obese and non-obese persons across groups. The table has m rows and two columns, and each cell of the table contains the observed number of persons in that group.
4. Create the corresponding table for the predicted number of persons in each group, where the predicted number is given by the sum of the predicted probabilities in that group.

5. Compare the observed and predicted numbers in corresponding cells in the two tables. If they are close, the model is well calibrated.

A statistical way to compare observed and predicted quantities is to look at the standardized difference between them. This can be done by calculating the difference between observed and predicted numbers in each cell, scaled by the square root of the predicted numbers. For contingency tables, this is known as *Pearson's residual*:

$$\text{Res} = \frac{\text{Observed} - \text{Predicted}}{\sqrt{\text{Predicted}}}.$$

Pearson's residual tells us about overprediction and underprediction within each cell of the table. To summarize across groups, Hosmer and Lemeshow suggest summing the square of the Pearson's residuals (Res^2) over the table and comparing it to a χ^2 ("chi-squared") distribution with $m - 2$ degrees of freedom.

The Hosmer–Lemeshow χ^2 test can be problematic for large sample sizes because it can reject models that approximate the data reasonably well but not perfectly. A simulation study suggested not using the test when sample size is larger than 10,000 and to use more than $m = 100$ groups for sample sizes around 5000 [8]. Still, partitioning the data into few groups (say $m = 10$ or 20) and looking for cells with relatively extreme residuals can be a useful informal tool for model checking. Any systematic pattern of residuals across the cells can be informative about the validity of linearity assumptions or may suggest a need to include additional covariates.

Table 4.6 shows observed and predicted numbers of obese and non-obese persons in $m = 10$ groups. The Pearson's residuals are distributed across groups without patterns or extreme values. However, the Hosmer–Lemeshow statistic is calculated to be 21.1, corresponding to a p-value of 0.007 according to a χ^2 with 8 degrees

Table 4.6 Observed (Obs) and predicted (Pred) numbers of obese and non-obese persons by decile of predicted probabilities and corresponding Pearson's residuals (Res) based on the model in Table 4.5

Group	$\text{Obs}_{\text{obese}}$	$\text{Obs}_{\text{non-obese}}$	$\text{Pred}_{\text{obese}}$	$\text{Pred}_{\text{non-obese}}$	$\text{Res}_{\text{obese}}$	$\text{Res}_{\text{non-obese}}$
1	148	479	123.7	503.3	2.2	−1.1
2	147	512	169.1	489.9	−1.7	1.0
3	188	460	187.5	460.5	0.0	−0.0
4	197	447	207.5	436.5	−0.7	0.5
5	227	417	227.9	416.1	−0.1	0.0
6	215	426	242.9	398.1	−1.8	1.4
7	281	360	262.4	378.6	1.2	−1.0
8	295	351	289.3	356.7	0.3	−0.3
9	307	343	315.5	334.5	−0.5	0.5
10	378	269	357.3	289.7	1.1	−1.2

of freedom. If we partition the data into $m = 100$ groups, the p-value is 0.02. In both cases, we would conclude that the model was not well calibrated, but, given our sample size of over 6800 individuals, would take this result with a grain of salt.

What is the Hosmer–Lemeshow test actually evaluating? It is sometimes billed as a check on the linearity assumption of the logistic regression model. But really it is an omnibus test of the ability of the model to replicate the pattern of $Y = 1$ and $Y = 0$ across groups of observations given the covariates included and the structure of the model. If there is a specific concern that an important covariate may have been omitted or that a polynomial or interaction term should be added, this can be explicitly examined via likelihood-based statistics such as the AIC and BIC discussed above.

4.7.3 Model Prediction: ROC and AUC

If the objective of the analysis is prediction, measures of predictive accuracy are most relevant. By *prediction*, we mean an educated guess about a future outcome based on the values of relevant covariates. In the case of binary outcomes, there are several standard measures of predictive accuracy.

A simple way to think about the predictive accuracy of a binary regression model is to look at the overlap between the distributions of the predicted probabilities for positive and negative observed outcomes. Figure 4.5 shows histograms of predicted probabilities for obese and non-obese persons. While the predicted probabilities tend to be lower for non-obese persons than for obese persons, there is considerable overlap between the two histograms, illustrating relatively weak discrimination between these two groups.

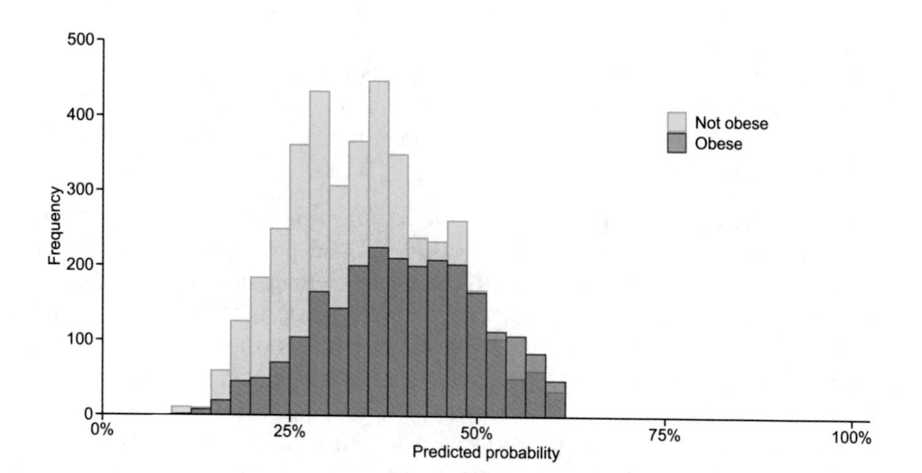

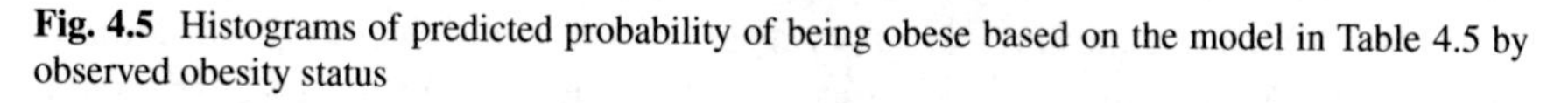

Fig. 4.5 Histograms of predicted probability of being obese based on the model in Table 4.5 by observed obesity status

Table 4.7 Frequency of observed (Obs) and predicted (Pred) obese and non-obese persons based on the model in Table 4.5 using a threshold of $T = 0.5$ for predictions

Status	$\text{Pred}_{\text{non-obese}}$	$\text{Pred}_{\text{obese}}$	Total
$\text{Obs}_{\text{non-obese}}$	3740 (92.0%)	324 (8.0%)	4064 (100.0%)
$\text{Obs}_{\text{obese}}$	1950 (81.8%)	433 (18.2%)	2383 (100.0%)

Formal measures of predictive accuracy effectively quantify the agreement between the observed binary outcome and the model prediction. The model prediction is not binary; it is a probability between zero and one. But if one is willing to specify a threshold T above which a prediction is positive (one) and below which a prediction is negative (zero), then one could assess agreement between the observed binary outcome and the binarized predicted outcome.

A natural threshold is $T = 0.5$, where a person is predicted to be positive ($Y = 1$) if the predicted probability is greater than 0.5 and he/she is predicted to be negative ($Y = 0$) otherwise. Table 4.7 presents the results of this approach for the multivariate logistic regression in Table 4.5. The rows of this two-way table show the observed obesity status, and the columns show predicted obesity status based on the threshold $T = 0.5$. We see that 92% of non-obese persons are correctly predicted to be non-obese by this model and this criterion, but only 18% of obese persons are correctly predicted to be obese. Correctly classifying obese persons may be more important than correctly classifying non-obese persons, and this can be controlled by changing the threshold.

In the setting of binary outcomes, two basic measures of predictive accuracy play a central role:

Sensitivity: The probability that the model prediction is positive when the outcome is positive. Sensitivity measures the ability of the model to correctly predict a positive outcome. In the obesity example, for the threshold $T = 0.5$, the sensitivity is 18%.

Specificity: The probability that the model prediction is negative when the outcome is negative. Specificity measures the ability of the model to correctly predict a negative outcome. In the obesity example, for the threshold $T = 0.5$, the specificity is 92%.

The sensitivity is also referred to as the *true-positive rate* (TPR), while one minus the specificity is the *false-positive rate* (FPR). Good predictive performance is characterized by high TPR and low FPR, but in many settings, the importance of one outweighs that of the other. For example, in developing tests to diagnose COVID-19, high sensitivity is critical because infected individuals who test negative (false negative) may continue to spread the infection unwittingly. On the other hand, in developing tests to detect COVID-19 antibodies, high specificity is critical because individuals who have not had the virus but who think that they have had it (false positive) may behave as if they are protected when they are not.

It should be apparent that sensitivity and specificity will vary depending on the threshold T. As the threshold increases, the sensitivity will decrease but specificity

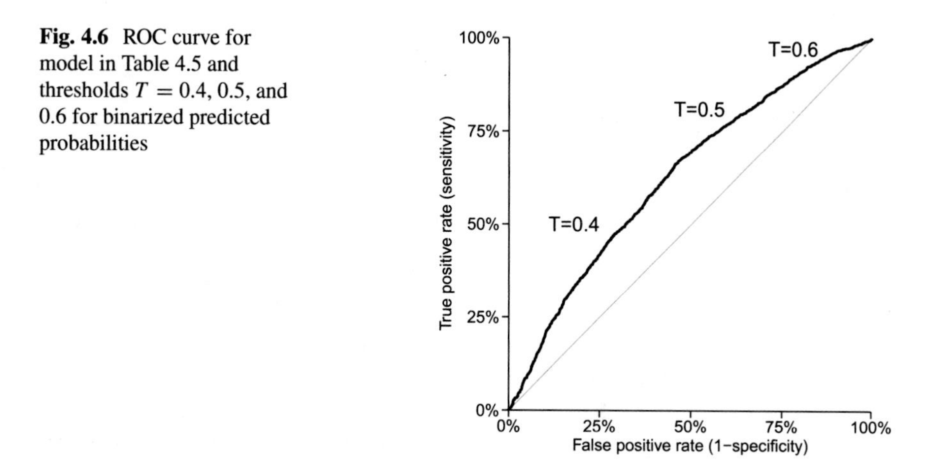

Fig. 4.6 ROC curve for model in Table 4.5 and thresholds $T = 0.4, 0.5$, and 0.6 for binarized predicted probabilities

will increase. Thus, sensitivity and specificity move in opposite directions as the threshold T varies. When choosing a specific threshold T to dichotomize predictions from a binary regression model, it is important to consider the consequences of both false negatives and false positives and to weight them appropriately in the selection of T. However, generally speaking, we would like to judge predictive accuracy without specifying a threshold. The *receiver operating characteristic* (ROC) curve does this.

The ROC curve plots the TPR (sensitivity) versus the FPR ($1 -$ specificity) as T varies. Figure 4.6 considers the problem of predicting obesity based on the model in Table 4.5. Naturally, if we really wanted to predict whether a person was obese or would become obese, we would bring many more covariates to bear. But for illustration, we plot the ROC curve for this model. T increases from zero to one; both the TPR (sensitivity) and FPR ($1 -$ specificity) increase from zero to one. The ideal ROC curve hugs the upper left corner of the unit square, where the TPR is highest and the FPR is lowest.

A quantitative measure of the predictive performance of an ROC curve is the *area under the curve* (AUC), sometimes also called the *concordance* or *C-statistic*. The ideal ROC curve has an AUC of 1. An ROC curve that sits on the 45-degree line that bisects the unit square reflects predictive accuracy that is no better than flipping a coin; it has an AUC of 0.5. For the multivariate regression in Table 4.5, the ROC is only somewhat above the 45 degree line, and the AUC is a relatively unimpressive 0.63. Incorporating other variables in the model, such as chronic conditions (e.g., diabetes, hypertension, and cardiovascular disease), behaviors like exercise, and socioeconomic factors like income and education, might improve the predictive performance. We discuss models for analyses in which accurate prediction is the objective in Chap. 10.

4.8 Multinomial Regression

4.8.1 An Extension of Logistic Regression

Multinomial regression extends logistic regression to settings where the outcome variable has more than two categories. To illustrate, we examine how SEX, RACE, AGE, and YEAR are associated with the probability of four BMI categories: underweight (BMI $<$ 18.5), normal (18.5 $\leq$ BMI $<$ 25), overweight (25 $\leq$ BMI $<$ 30), and obese (BMI $\geq$ 30). Multinomial regression translates this question into how the covariates are associated with observed proportions in these categories. In principle, we could repeat the logistic regression analysis in Table 4.5 for each BMI category separately. However, such an analysis ignores important aspects of the multi-category setting. We will compare the two approaches and discuss the differences between them.

We start this section with a single binary covariate, YEAR. Table 4.8 shows frequencies within the different BMI categories in 1999–2000 and 2015–2016. The absolute 8% increase in the obese category coincided with an absolute decrease of 5% in the normal category and an absolute decrease of 3% in the overweight category. The proportions of underweight persons were small and similar in absolute magnitude in the 2 survey years. The risk ratios (RRs) and odds ratios (ORs) summarize relative change between years, but these measures do not take the multi-category structure into account.

First we define a multi-category OR of category k relative to a reference category as:

$$\text{OR} = \frac{P(Y = k \mid 2015\text{–}2016)/P(Y = \text{reference} \mid 2015\text{–}2016)}{P(Y = k \mid 1999\text{–}2000)/P(Y = \text{reference} \mid 1999\text{–}2000)}.$$

This definition of OR extends the one for binary outcomes for which the relative category was always $Y = 0$. The bottom row of Table 4.8 shows the multi-category ORs taking normal weight as the reference category. These multi-category ORs could be obtained by calculating two-category ORs from two-way tables of each category with the reference category. For example, the multi-category OR of 1.07

Table 4.8 Frequency of persons in BMI categories age 20–59 years in NHANES sample data for 1999–2000 and 2015–2016 and measures of relative change

Year	Underweight	Normal	Overweight	Obese
1999–2000	49 (1.7%)	920 (32.7%)	930 (33.1%)	914 (32.5%)
2015–2016	57 (1.6%)	1013 (27.9%)	1095 (30.1%)	1469 (40.4%)
Difference	−0.00	−0.05	−0.03	0.08
Risk ratio	0.90	0.85	0.91	1.24
Odds ratio	0.90	0.80	0.87	1.41
Multi-category OR	1.06	1.00	1.07	1.46

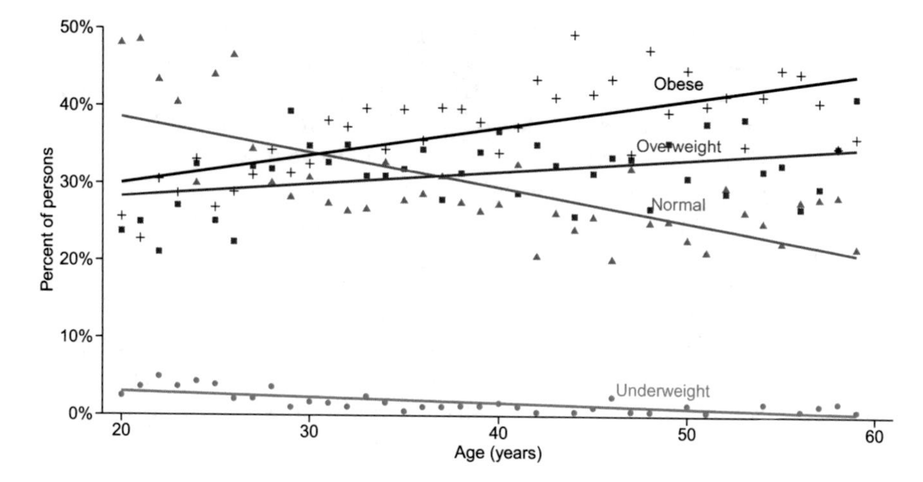

Fig. 4.7 Percent of persons age 20–59 years in BMI categories in NHANES sample data in 1999–2000 and 2015–2016 with separate linear regressions

for overweight persons is the two-category OR based on the normal and overweight columns in Table 4.8, which can be calculated as $(920 \times 1095)/(930 \times 1013)$.

Based on the multi-category OR, we estimate a 6% increase in the odds of being underweight, a 7% increase in the odds of being overweight, and a 46% increase in the odds of being obese relative to the change in normal weight persons in 2015–2016 compared to 1999–2000. Thus, the multi-category ORs characterize the relative change within each category relative to the change in the reference category.

For further comparison with the binary case, Fig. 4.7 shows the proportions of persons in each BMI category by age. The points show the observed proportions, and the lines are separate linear regressions for each category.

We introduced binary regression out of concerns about predictions that are outside the sensible [0, 1] range and the non-normal distribution of binary outcomes. For multinomial outcomes, an additional consideration is that predictions across categories should sum to 1 at each age—and, more generally, at each value of the covariates. Multinomial regression is precisely designed for this purpose. For each subject, multinomial regression predicts the probability that they belong to each category in a way that respects the multi-category nature of the outcome.

In both binary and multinomial regressions, the central question is whether and how the proportions of the outcome variable change with the covariates. Whether the outcome variable has two, three, or more categories, addressing this question involves assessing the shape of the outcome distribution given the covariates. In the case of a binary outcome, the overall proportions are $p_0 = P(Y = 0)$ and $p_1 = P(Y = 1)$. In the case of a multinomial outcome with three categories, the overall proportions are $p_0 = P(Y = 0)$, $p_1 = P(Y = 1)$, and $p_2 = P(Y = 2)$. In general, for K categories, the overall proportions are $p_0 = P(Y = 0)$, $p_1 = P(Y = 1)$, $p_2 = P(Y = 2), \ldots, p_{K-1} = P(Y = K - 1)$.

Binary regression addresses the central question by examining how the ratio p_1/p_0, the odds of a positive outcome, depends on the covariates. Testing whether the odds of Y changes as X changes from 0 to 1 is equivalent to testing whether the outcome distribution changes. In the case of a binary covariate, the OR is the ratio of the odds (of a positive outcome) when $X = 1$ compared to when $X = 0$.

In the case of a K-category outcome, multinomial regression examines $K - 1$ ratios, $p_1/p_0, p_2/p_0, \ldots, p_{K-1}/p_0$. As in binary regression, testing whether any of these ratios changes as X changes from 0 to 1 is equivalent to testing whether the outcome distribution changes. Multinomial regression analysis therefore consists of multiple regressions, each one corresponding to one of these ratios.

In our example of $K = 4$ BMI categories, $p_0 = P(Y = \text{normal})$, $p_1 = P(Y = \text{underweight})$, $p_2 = P(Y = \text{overweight})$, and $p_3 = P(Y = \text{obese})$, and there are three regression models to fit, each of which is similar to the logistic regression in Eq. (4.2):

$$\log(p_1/p_0) = \beta_0 + \beta_1 X$$
$$\log(p_2/p_0) = \gamma_0 + \gamma_1 X$$
$$\log(p_3/p_0) = \delta_0 + \delta_1 X.$$

Note that each model has its own set of parameters and, moreover, the covariates can vary across models. However, the odds in the three models share the same reference category ($Y = 0$). In each model, the coefficient of X can be interpreted as the log of a quantity analogous to an OR. In the first model, this quantity is the ratio p_1/p_0 when $X = 1$ divided by the ratio p_1/p_0 when $X = 0$. This is sometimes referred to as a *relative risk ratio*, but for consistency with the binary case, we will continue to refer to it as an OR.

If the OR is greater than 1, corresponding to $\beta_1 > 0$, this means that an increase in X from 0 to 1 corresponds to a shift in the proportion of the outcome in category $Y = 0$ into category $Y = 1$. Similarly, if the OR in the second regression is greater than 1, corresponding to $\gamma_1 > 0$, this means that an increase in X from 0 to 1 corresponds to a shift in the proportion of the outcome in category $Y = 0$ into category $Y = 2$. We fit only three regressions for our four-category variable because the fourth category is completely determined by the first three.

Table 4.9 compares separate logistic regressions to multinomial regression. For example, the logistic regression for obese persons was fit using only data for obese and normal weight persons after removing underweight and overweight persons. It is therefore different from the logistic regression in Table 4.5, which was fit using underweight, normal and overweight as "non-obese" persons. The coefficients in the separate logistic regression and the joint multinomial regression are almost identical; the two sets of results give similar insights into the data. For example, the coefficients for YEAR = 2015–2016 are all positive; equivalently, the ORs are greater than 1, indicating that the odds of each "non-normal" BMI category relative to the normal category were higher in 2015–2016.

Table 4.9 Separate logistic regressions (LR) and multinomial regression (MR) of BMI categories for persons age 20–59 years in NHANES sample data for 1999–2000 and 2015–2016

Category	Predictor	Coef. (LR)	SE (LR)	P (LR)	OR (LR)	Coef. (MR)	SE (MR)	P (MR)	OR (MR)
Underweight	Intercept	−2.44	0.25	<0.001	0.09	−2.42	0.25	<0.001	0.09
	SEX = Female	0.39	0.21	0.07	1.47	0.39	0.21	0.06	1.48
	RACE = Non-Hispanic black	−0.45	0.30	0.13	0.64	−0.47	0.29	0.11	0.63
	RACE = Mexican American	−0.61	0.32	0.06	0.54	−0.60	0.32	0.06	0.55
	RACE = Other Hispanic	−0.27	0.38	0.5	0.76	−0.23	0.37	0.5	0.79
	RACE = Other/mixed	−0.35	0.30	0.3	0.71	−0.40	0.30	0.18	0.67
	AGE	−0.03	0.01	<0.001	0.97	−0.04	0.01	<0.001	0.96
	YEAR = 2015–2016	0.12	0.21	0.6	1.12	0.15	0.21	0.5	1.16
Overweight	Intercept	−0.35	0.09	<0.001	0.71	−0.34	0.09	<0.001	0.71
	SEX = Female	−0.35	0.07	<0.001	0.71	−0.35	0.06	<0.001	0.70
	RACE = Non-Hispanic black	0.02	0.09	0.8	1.02	0.04	0.09	0.6	1.04
	RACE = Mexican American	0.54	0.09	<0.001	1.72	0.54	0.09	<0.001	1.72
	RACE = Other Hispanic	0.40	0.12	<0.001	1.50	0.42	0.12	<0.001	1.52
	RACE = Other/mixed	−0.56	0.11	<0.001	0.57	−0.51	0.11	<0.001	0.60
	AGE	0.02	0.00	<0.001	1.02	0.02	0.00	<0.001	1.02
	YEAR = 2015–2016	0.20	0.07	0.003	1.23	0.16	0.07	0.02	1.18
Obese	Intercept	−0.89	0.09	<0.001	0.41	−0.89	0.09	<0.001	0.41
	SEX = Female	0.22	0.06	<0.001	1.25	0.22	0.06	<0.001	1.25
	RACE = Non-Hispanic black	0.49	0.09	<0.001	1.64	0.48	0.09	<0.001	1.61
	RACE = Mexican American	0.69	0.09	<0.001	1.99	0.67	0.09	<0.001	1.95
	RACE = Other Hispanic	0.46	0.12	<0.001	1.58	0.46	0.12	<0.001	1.58
	RACE = Other/mixed	−0.87	0.11	<0.001	0.42	−0.88	0.11	<0.001	0.42
	AGE	0.03	0.00	<0.001	1.03	0.03	0.00	<0.001	1.03
	YEAR = 2015–2016	0.51	0.07	<0.001	1.67	0.52	0.07	<0.001	1.69

For a more specific interpretation of these results, consider the multi-category ORs from the multinomial regression, which (like the ORs in the logistic regressions) are just the exponentiated coefficients. The ORs for YEAR = 2015–2016 for the underweight and overweight categories are 1.16 and 1.18, which means that from 1999–2000 to 2015–2016, the estimated probability of each of these categories relative to the normal BMI category increased by 16% and 18%. The OR for the obese category is much larger (1.69), showing a larger relative shift into that category between the years.

In summary, interpretation of multinomial regression results is similar to the interpretation of logistic regression results when data are restricted to only two categories. The effects of the covariates may differ from category to category and may be positive for one category and negative for another. For example, age has a significant negative effect for underweight persons, meaning that older people have lower odds of being underweight than younger people (in the age range considered). However, age has a significant positive effect for overweight and obese persons, meaning that older people have higher odds of being in these groups than younger people (in the age range considered).

4.8.2 Marginal Effects

If there are K categories in the outcome, multinomial regression runs $K - 1$ regressions and yields $K - 1$ sets of coefficients to interpret. This can get cumbersome quite quickly; moreover, it can be difficult to make inferences about how the overall shape of the outcome distribution changes based on the estimated relative risk ratios.

A *recycled predictions* approach can be used to obtain inferences on the original probability scale of the outcome variable. For the YEAR variable, this works by calculating the predicted probabilities of each of the four categories of BMI for each person, first setting their YEAR to 1999–2000 and then to 2015–2016. This produces two sets of four numbers with predicted probabilities in either set that sum to 1. The four numbers are then averaged across individuals in the sample, and then the difference in averages between sets is calculated to produce a *marginal additive effect* on the probability scale. This exactly replicates the method used for logistic regression. The marginal additive effect is the difference in average predicted values for each BMI category and reflects the estimated change in the probability of being in that BMI category between years.

Table 4.10 shows the recycled prediction estimates of the marginal additive effect of YEAR on the probability of being in each BMI category. The columns show the average predicted probability of being in each BMI category under the estimated model if all persons were in the indicated survey year. The last column shows the difference in 2015–2016 relative to 1999–2000. The results indicate that the more recent survey year is associated with a nearly 10% increase in the probability of being in the obese category. This increase in the obese category corresponds to

Table 4.10 The marginal additive effect of YEAR calculated as the mean difference of predicted probabilities if all persons were in the indicated BMI category in 1999–2000 and in 2015–2016 based on the multinomial model in Table 4.9

Category	YEAR = 1999–2000	YEAR = 2015–2016	Marginal additive effect
Underweight	0.017	0.016	−0.001
Normal	0.339	0.269	−0.070
Overweight	0.328	0.302	−0.026
Obese	0.316	0.413	0.097

decreases of 7% in the normal and of 3% in the overweight categories. There is virtually no change in the underweight category.

4.8.3 Ordered Multinomial Regression

Multinomial regression is sometimes referred to as an "unordered" multinomial logit model, because it is agnostic to any implied ordering of the categories. When categories have an ordering, such as BMI categories, or self-reported health status, another multi-category regression model is also available. It makes fairly strong assumptions, so we do not generally recommend its use; however, it is widely available, so we briefly summarize its structure and limitations.

The *proportional odds model* [9] is derived assuming that the categories reflect intervals partitioning an underlying continuous scale. Like the multinomial model, the proportional odds model includes a set of logit-type regression equations. For Y = BMI and X = YEAR, the equations can be written:

$$\text{logit}[P(Y > k)] = \gamma_k + \beta X,$$

for $k = 1$ to $K - 1$, where $K = 4$ is the number of BMI categories. Thus, this model describes how the log odds of being in a higher category relative to being in a lower one depend on covariates. When $X = 0$, the coefficients γ_k describe the multinomial probability distribution of BMI categories in 1999–2000. When $X = 1$, the distribution of BMI is allowed to change but only in a highly restrictive, monotone way because there is only one coefficient, β, describing this change.

If β is positive, then the log odds of being in a higher BMI category increases in the later year, and this increase is the same regardless of the specific category. Thus, the log odds of being overweight or higher and the log odds of being obese both increase by the same amount from 1999–2000 to 2015–2016. On the probability scale, we have probability shifting from lower categories to higher categories in a manner prescribed by β. But this monotone constraint does not accommodate a variety of association patterns. For example, if X is a binary version of an extended age variable that includes all ages, we might find that both overweight and underweight increase for elderly individuals. This kind of pattern, where multinomial probabilities become weighted toward extreme categories as a covariate changes values, would not be possible to model or detect with a proportional odds model, but it would be identified with an unordered multinomial logit model. Therefore, we generally recommend the unordered model unless a specific hypothesis that conforms with the assumptions of proportional odds is of particular interest.

4.9 Software and Data

R code to download data and to carry out the examples in this book is available at the GitHub page https://roman-gulati.github.io/statistics-for-health-data-science/. In addition to the R packages cited in Chap. 1, this chapter also used the `pROC` [10] and `margins` [5] packages.

References

1. Pettiti, D.B.: Associations are not effects. Am. J. Epidemiol. **133**(2), 101–102 (1991)
2. Schulman, K.A., Berlin, J.A., Harless, W., Kerner, J.F., Sistrunk, S., Gersh, B.J., Dubé, R., Taleghani, C.K., Burke, J.E., Williams, S., Eisenberg, J.M., Ayers, W., Escarce, J.J.: The effect of race and sex on physicians' recommendations for cardiac catheterization. N. Engl. J. Med. **340**(8), 618–626 (1999)
3. Schwartz, L.M., Woloshin, S., Welch, H.G.: Misunderstandings about the effects of race and sex on physicians' referrals for cardiac catheterization. N. Engl. J. Med. **341**(4), 279–283 (1999)
4. Kleinman, L.C., Norton, E.C.: What's the risk? A simple approach for estimating adjusted risk measures from nonlinear models including logistic regression. Health Serv. Res. **44**(1), 288–302 (2009)
5. Leeper, T.J.: margins: Marginal effects for model objects. R package version 0.3.23 (2018)
6. Zou, G.: A modified Poisson regression approach to prospective studies with binary data. Am. J. Epidemiol. **159**(7), 702–706 (2004)
7. Hosmer, D.W., Lemeshow, S.: Goodness of fit tests for the multiple logistic regression model. Comput. Stat. Theory Methods **9**(10), 1043–1069 (1980)
8. Paul, P., Pennell, M.L., Lemeshow, S.: Standardizing the power of the Hosmer-Lemeshow goodness of fit test in large data sets. Stat. Med. **32**(1), 67–80 (2013)
9. McCullagh, P.: Regression models for ordinal data. J. R. Stat. Soc. Ser. B **42**, 109–142 (1980)
10. Robin, X., Turck, N., Hainard, A., Tiberti, N., Lisacek, F., Sanchez, J.C., Müller, M.: pROC: An open-source package for R and S+ to analyze and compare ROC curves. BMC Bioinf. **12**, 77 (2011)

Chapter 5
Count Outcomes

Abstract This chapter addresses the analysis of count outcomes, which are common in the study of health care utilization. Examples include the number of hospitalizations, diagnostic tests, or outpatient visits within a specified period of observation. Count outcomes are also common in the setting of health surveillance, where annual counts of disease cases or deaths are critically important in measuring spatial or temporal trends and monitoring for unexpected outbreaks. Poisson regression provides a framework for studying correlates of count outcomes, but this framework can be limiting and does not capture the overdispersion that is characteristic of most observational health care datasets. Negative binomial regression provides an alternative that is often preferred in practice. We describe both approaches in detail and show how negative binomial regression naturally extends the Poisson framework to a setting that reflects between-individual heterogeneity. Generalized linear models (GLMs) provide a unifying framework that includes these models as special cases. We conclude the chapter with a discussion of the GLM framework, its place in the development of the science and art of statistical regression methods, and its utility to the health data analyst.

5.1 Count Outcomes

A count outcome reflects a cumulative process in which events are tallied to produce the reported result. The process can occur over time (e.g., number of hospitalizations or medical visits for an individual), over space (e.g., number of animals of a particular species within areas of a given size), or over people (e.g., number of cancer cases in a population). Count data have unique properties that require special modeling approaches, and this chapter provides an introduction to the most commonly used ones.

We begin by reviewing key aspects of the linear regression model for a continuous outcome (see Chap. 3). The model was presented as having two parts: a systematic part that defines the mean of the outcome as a deterministic function of predictors and a random part that adds error, or noise, around its mean. This enables

R. Etzioni et al., *Statistics for Health Data Science*, Springer Texts in Statistics,
https://doi.org/10.1007/978-3-030-59889-1_5

separate modeling assumptions for the mean (linearity) and for the spread around it (constant variance).

When analyzing count data, the separation of systematic and random parts is rarely possible. Indeed, it is generally the case that the spread around the mean increases as the mean increases. There are two major approaches for tackling this problem. The first assumes a parametric distribution for the data that encodes a mean–variance relationship, the most basic being a Poisson distribution, and fits a regression to the mean of this distribution. The specific distribution assumed explicitly determines the variance given the mean, but this assumption exposes the analysis to potential problems of model mis-specification. The second approach uses quasilikelihood methods to model the variance as a function of the mean without specifying a distribution. We focus on parametric models; for further reading about the quasilikelihood approach, see McCullagh and Nelder [1].

5.2 The Poisson Distribution

When the accumulation process is highly regular, the resulting count can be described using one of a handful of statistical distributions, the most well-known being the Poisson distribution. We begin by defining what is meant by highly regular and introduce the Poisson distribution in the context of events accumulating over a time interval. Consider an event-generating process with the following properties:

(1) The probability of at least one event in a very small interval is proportional to the length of that interval.
(2) The probability that two or more occurrences of the event in a very small interval is negligible.
(3) The numbers of events in nonoverlapping intervals are mutually independent of one another.

In other words, events occur independently of one another, one at a time, and at a constant rate. These properties determine a general type of process that is not necessarily limited to events over time. For example, events could occur over a small area or volume of space or to individual persons in a population. In the population setting, properties (1)–(3) imply that the probability of the event of interest (e.g., the diagnosis of a certain disease) is very small and that individuals are independent.

When considering events over time, a direct consequence of properties (1)–(3) is that the resulting process is *memoryless*, meaning that the chance that an event will occur within an interval beginning at time t does not depend on what happened before t. For example, if no events have occurred for a long time before t, this does not imply that one can expect that an event is imminent.

The memoryless property is violated when the occurrence of an event precludes another event. For example, this property is violated if an outpatient visit, the event of interest, leads to a hospital stay during which, by definition, outpatient

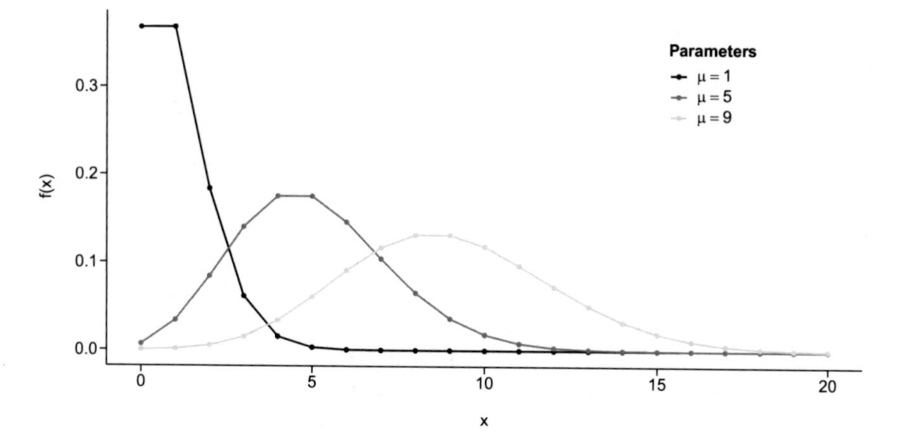

Fig. 5.1 Poisson probability density functions for different values of the mean μ

visits cannot occur or if a prescription refill, the event of interest, precludes reimbursement for a period of time during which further prescription refills cannot occur. Nonetheless, it is helpful to first model the simple setting in which properties (1)–(3) hold before moving on to more complex event-generating processes.

In the highly regular setting defined by properties (1)–(3), the number of events in an interval of observation has a Poisson distribution, and the expected number of events is simply given by the rate of events per unit time multiplied by the length of the interval. For example, if outpatient visits occur, on average, once per month, then the expected number of outpatient visits in a year is 12.

Figure 5.1 shows a few Poisson distributions with different means. The figure shows that the mean of the distribution defines not only its location but also its shape and spread. The variance of a Poisson distribution is equal to its mean, so that as the expected number of events per unit time increases, so does the variability, according to a tightly prescribed relationship.

5.3 Two Count Data Regression Models

We use two examples to illustrate the development and application of count data regression models. In the first model, the outcome variable is the number of outpatient visits in a specified interval, and in the second model, the outcome variable is the number of cancer deaths in a specified population.

5.3.1 Modeling Health Care Utilization

The first example is a historic study of health care utilization among participants in a subsidized health insurance plan of low-income individuals in Washington State. The Basic Health Plan (BHP) of Washington State was a pilot project to provide health care benefits for uninsured, low-income families (i.e., income below twice the Federal poverty line). The plan contracted with managed health care systems to provide subsidized basic health services and studied health care utilization and outcomes across the systems involved. Martin et al. [2] provide a detailed description of the BHP and its objectives.

We use data from three counties that participated in the plan, namely, Spokane, Pierce, and Clallam counties. Both Spokane and Pierce counties include a metropolitan area, whereas Clallam is more rural. In Spokane, care was provided by an existing health maintenance organization (HMO) with 22 salaried primary care physicians who made referrals to specialists. In Pierce and Clallam, care was provided by an existing independent practice association (IPA) sponsored by the county physicians' bureau. Spokane later added an IPA option, and thus we analyze data pertaining to four providers across the three counties. Since participants in the BHP had previously been uninsured, a key research question addresses patterns of health care utilization among a "newly insured" population. Martin et al. [2] provide an analysis specifically addressing this question. Here we use count data modeling to examine outpatient visits and to compare the frequency of visits across the four providers.

5.3.2 Modeling Mortality in a Cancer Registry

Our second example of the use of count data models is a disease surveillance problem. We examine annual prostate cancer mortality rates among black and white men using population cancer registry data from the Surveillance, Epidemiology, and End Results (SEER) registry of US National Cancer Institute [3]. Since 1975, the SEER registry has ascertained information about cancer diagnosis and survival on all cases diagnosed within the registry's catchment areas. Prostate cancer is the most common cancer and the second leading cause of cancer death in US men [4].

The prostate cancer death rate among black men in the United States has historically been approximately double that among white men for reasons which remain unclear but are likely due to a combination of poorer access to care and potentially also biological differences in the disease by race. In the early 1990s, screening for prostate cancer using a simple blood test for prostate-specific antigen concentration became widespread in the United States. Since that time, disease mortality rates among both blacks and whites have been declining steadily. We use count data modeling to investigate whether the decline in death rates among black men matches that among white men.

5.4 Poisson Regression for Individual-Level Counts

Poisson regression is a framework for relating the mean of a count variable Y to predictors X. In the BHP example, a primary analytic objective is to compare outpatient visits (the outcome Y) across the four health care providers, taking into account differences in enrolled patients' characteristics. Table 5.1 gives the mean and standard deviation of individual outpatient visits across providers along with summary statistics for important predictors: duration of enrollment in months, age, sex, race, and number of chronic conditions. It is clear that the Spokane IPA, which was incorporated into the BHP later than the other programs, has the lowest mean outpatient visits but also the lowest mean enrollment duration.

Figure 5.2 plots the mean number of outpatient visits (Y) and the standard deviation of outpatient visits for the four providers (a predictor X). The number of outpatient visits is clearly more variable for providers with higher means. This pattern violates a key assumption needed for valid inference using standard linear regression—namely, that the variance is similar in all subgroups defined by the predictors.

There are other reasons to consider alternatives to linear regression. A count outcome can only take on nonnegative values, but linear regression is defined over the entire real line. We need a regression framework that focuses on the nonnegative real line so that we don't inadvertently find ourselves predicting negative count outcomes. In addition, the restriction of the outcome to integer values makes it

Table 5.1 Descriptive statistics of the Basic Health Plan data for persons age 18 years or older by health care provider

Characteristic	Spokane HMO	Spokane IPA	Pierce	Clallam
n	978	547	1641	521
Visits (mean (SD))	5.77 (11.23)	3.64 (4.84)	5.61 (8.10)	4.29 (5.49)
Enrollment (mean (SD))	23.87 (12.11)	16.45 (5.92)	22.69 (13.19)	21.10 (8.98)
Age (mean (SD))	38.43 (11.55)	37.02 (11.65)	35.75 (11.43)	37.58 (11.65)
Sex = Men (%)	382 (39.1)	216 (39.5)	586 (35.7)	214 (41.1)
Race (%)				
White	910 (93.0)	508 (92.9)	1403 (85.5)	484 (92.9)
Other	51 (5.2)	27 (4.9)	186 (11.3)	22 (4.2)
Unknown	17 (1.7)	12 (2.2)	52 (3.2)	15 (2.9)
Conditions (%)				
0	270 (27.6)	168 (30.7)	520 (31.7)	168 (32.2)
1	249 (25.5)	129 (23.6)	378 (23.0)	126 (24.2)
2	158 (16.2)	88 (16.1)	241 (14.7)	82 (15.7)
3	82 (8.4)	49 (9.0)	150 (9.1)	56 (10.7)
4	129 (13.2)	62 (11.3)	181 (11.0)	48 (9.2)
Unknown	90 (9.2)	51 (9.3)	171 (10.4)	41 (7.9)

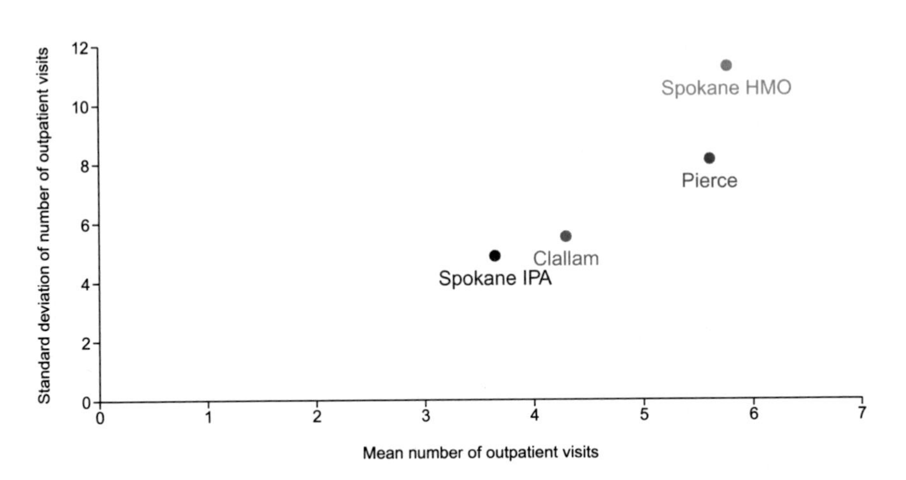

Fig. 5.2 Mean versus standard deviation of the number of outpatient visits in the Basic Health Plan by provider

almost impossible to model the errors around the regression line, suggesting that a different approach is needed.

Poisson regression achieves these objectives by positing a linear regression model for the log-transformed mean, $\log[E(Y)]$, and assuming a Poisson distribution for the outcome, rather than a model for the error terms.

The Poisson regression model imposes three assumptions. First, the outcome Y_i (e.g., outpatient visits) for subject i has a Poisson distribution with mean μ_i. Second, the mean μ_i of subject i depends on a set of k predictors, $X_{1i}, \ldots, X_{ki}$ (e.g., age and provider), so that individuals with exactly the same predictor values have exactly the same mean. And third, the mean outcome is related to the predictors via a log-linear model, which means that the log of the mean of the count response, Y_i, is a linear combination of the predictor variables:

$$\log(\mu_i) = \beta_0 + \beta_1 X_{1i} + \cdots + \beta_k X_{ki}.$$

This model allows the range of values on the right-hand side to span the entire real line while ensuring that $\mu_i = E(Y_i)$ is nonnegative because it is obtained by exponentiating the right-hand side:

$$\mu_i = \exp(\beta_0 + \beta_1 X_{1i} + \cdots + \beta_k X_{ki}).$$

Naturally, log-transforming the mean affects the interpretation of the coefficients. Specifically, a linear model for $\log(\mu)$ corresponds to a multiplicative model for μ. A one-unit change in predictor X_j corresponds to a multiplicative or *relative* effect of magnitude $\exp(\beta_j)$ on the mean of Y, often referred to as a relative risk. If there is no association between the predictor and $E(Y)$, then the relative risk will be close to 1.

Table 5.2 Fitted Poisson regression of outpatient visits in the Basic Health Plan adjusted for age, sex, race, and number of chronic conditions. Estimated risks are relative to Spokane HMO

Provider	Coefficient	Relative risk	95% CI	P-value
Spokane IPA	−0.33	0.72	(0.68, 0.76)	<0.001
Pierce	0.13	1.14	(1.10, 1.18)	<0.001
Clallam	−0.15	0.86	(0.82, 0.91)	<0.001

Let's now examine the coefficients and interpret them in the BHP example. Table 5.2 shows the results of a Poisson regression of outpatient visits in the BHP data. The hypothesis of interest is whether the mean number of visits differs across providers. Focusing on predisposing and need variables from the Anderson–Newman model of health care utilization described in Chap. 1, the model also adjusts for age (as a continuous variable), sex, an indicator of race group (white or others), and a count of chronic conditions at the time of enrollment (0, 1, 2, 3, 4, or more). The four-level categorical provider variable is entered using three binary dummy variables with reference category the Spokane HMO. The table provides the coefficient estimates as well as their exponentiated values.

The results quantify the multiplicative effect of provider relative to the Spokane HMO. Subjects in the Spokane IPA and Clallam programs are estimated to have had fewer visits on average, whereas subjects in Pierce county appear to have had more visits on average, than subjects in the Spokane HMO. The relative risk, $\exp(\beta)$, for Pierce is 1.14, which we interpret as indicating that the average number of outpatient visits among BHP subjects in Pierce county is 1.14 times or 14% higher than the average number in the Spokane HMO. In contrast, the average number of visits among BHP subjects in the Spokane IPA is 0.72 times or 28% lower than the average number among subjects in the Spokane HMO.

5.4.1 A Note on Multiplicative Versus Additive Effects

In Poisson regression, the natural interpretation of predictor effects is multiplicative; we make inferences about the relative risks or the percent increase or decrease in the mean of the count outcome. We are not restricted to this interpretation, however; if additive effects are of interest, they can be estimated by computing marginal additive effects using the technique of recycled predictions, described in Chap. 4.

Which metric is more appropriate, a multiplicative or an additive effect? In practice, the answer depends in large part on the scientific question. Scientific questions that relate to numbers or rates of events generally focus on multiplicative effects, expressing results in terms of relative risks. The relative risk is agnostic to the baseline frequency of the event; a relative risk of 1.5 (a 50% increase in risk) could mean that the expected number of events per unit time changed from 0.1 to 0.15 or from 10 to 15. In contrast, the additive effect, or risk difference, would be quite different in these two settings.

5.4.2 Accounting for Exposure

In a Poisson regression analysis, the duration over which count outcomes are ascertained is termed the *exposure*. Subjects with longer exposure have a greater opportunity to accumulate more events.

Table 5.1 provides the average duration of enrollment over which the outpatient visits accumulated in the BHP example calculated as the difference (in months) between each individual's date of enrollment into the BHP program until the date of analysis. The table shows that enrollment times were shorter on average in the Spokane IPA because its participants began later than participants covered by the other providers. Our finding of a lower average number of outpatient visits in the Spokane IPA was predicated on an implicit assumption that the enrollment duration was similar across individuals.

When the exposure is similar for all subjects in a count data analysis, then analyzing the number of events equates to analyzing the event intensity in terms of the rate per unit time (e.g., outpatient visits per month). However, when the exposure differs across subjects, then the number of events may misrepresent the event risk. Subjects with greater exposure may have more events recorded than subjects with lesser exposure simply because they have a greater opportunity to experience the event and not because they have a greater risk of the event.

To level the playing field when the exposure varies across subjects, we can model the average number of events per unit time rather than simply modeling the average number of events. This requires providing the regression model with a value for the count outcome as well as a value for the exposure associated with it. In the BHP example, we can scale the number of outpatient visits by the months enrolled and model the relationship between the monthly rate of visits and the predictor variables. Formally, if Y_i represents the number of events with mean μ_i and d_i is the months enrolled for subject i, then we can define $\lambda_i = \mu_i/d_i$ as the expected events per month for subject i. Modeling λ_i rather than μ_i leads to a more equitable comparison of the risk of the event of interest across the predictors.

With this change, our log-linear model becomes:

$$\log(\lambda_i) = \log(\mu_i/d_i) = \beta_0 + \beta_1 X_{1i} + \cdots + \beta_k X_{ki}.$$

Since $\log(\mu_i/d_i) = \log(\mu_i) - \log(d_i)$, this can be rewritten as:

$$\log(\mu_i) = \log(d_i) + \beta_0 + \beta_1 X_{1i} + \cdots + \beta_k X_{ki}.$$

Thus, the only difference between the model accounting for exposure time and the original model that didn't account for exposure time is the extra term, $\log(d_i)$, in the regression equation. This term is referred to as an *offset* because it is a known measurement with no associated coefficient. By including the exposure as an offset, the coefficients in this equation are interpretable as the effects of the predictors on the number of events per unit time rather than on the overall number of events.

Table 5.3 Fitted Poisson regression of outpatient visits in the Basic Health Plan including the exposure variable adjusted for age, sex, race, and number of chronic conditions. Estimated risks are relative to Spokane HMO

Provider	Coefficient	Relative risk	95% CI	*P*-value
Spokane IPA	0.04	1.04	(0.99, 1.10)	0.14
Pierce	0.13	1.14	(1.10, 1.18)	<0.001
Clallam	−0.03	0.97	(0.92, 1.02)	0.2

This is a key difference and one that may lead to completely different inferences regarding the predictors of interest. Making inference without taking into account differences in exposure time among individuals will lead to a biased result and incorrect conclusions.

In the case of the Basic Health Plan, the data include the enrollment duration for each individual. Table 5.3 shows results accounting for the exposure variable. Including the enrollment duration as an offset produces quite a different picture regarding the comparison of expected outpatient visits across providers. Indeed, the exponentiated coefficient estimate for the Spokane IPA turns out to be 1.04 in this model, which is not significantly different when compared with the Spokane HMO. We conclude that once we take exposure into account, there is no evidence that the frequency of outpatient visits differed between the Spokane HMO and the Spokane IPA programs.

5.5 Poisson Regression for Population Counts

We now turn to a different type of count data regression problem that is commonly encountered in surveillance research [e.g., 5]. In this setting, the outcome variable is the number of individuals experiencing the event, and the exposure is the size of the population eligible for the event. Poisson regression applied to annualized disease incidence and mortality counts is useful for making inferences about population trends over time in the burden of disease.

In cancer surveillance research, age–period–cohort (APC) modeling uses Poisson regression as a framework to learn about the links between cancer incidence and age, calendar period, and birth cohort [e.g., 6]. APC models for breast cancer identified prominent cohort effects due to changes in reproductive variables that correlated with birth year. Similar models applied to esophageal cancer identified strong period effects correlated with calendar trends in obesity. Our next example studies trends in prostate cancer mortality by race and uses Poisson regression to determine whether the trend is similar for black and white men in the United States.

Table 5.4 shows annual counts of prostate cancer deaths among white and black men in the nine original catchment areas of the SEER registry from 1990 to 2012 along with the population counts in these areas. The count outcome variable is annual prostate cancer deaths; the exposure is the population. There are 46

Table 5.4 Prostate cancer death rates for white (W) and black (B) men, 1990–2012

Year	Deaths (W)	Population (W)	Rate (W)	Deaths (B)	Population (B)	Rate (B)
1990	26,909	38,401,602	82.9	5175	3,907,099	181.1
1991	27,964	39,224,629	84.8	5294	4,030,248	181.7
1992	28,418	40,124,160	84.3	5482	4,163,129	185.5
1993	28,839	41,023,526	84.3	5655	4,296,920	190.2
1994	28,905	41,947,553	82.8	5646	4,443,336	185.8
1995	28,481	42,922,295	79.9	5589	4,599,961	181.7
1996	28,014	43,907,077	76.7	5714	4,762,692	183.2
1997	27,037	44,978,055	72.8	5462	4,944,660	172.6
1998	26,409	46,040,219	69.4	5434	5,127,708	169.1
1999	25,996	47,087,368	67.2	5356	5,315,503	163.0
2000	25,335	48,098,396	64.5	5344	5,511,155	160.1
2001	25,062	49,106,595	62.7	5264	5,695,002	157.6
2002	24,911	50,071,960	61.2	5143	5,877,088	151.0
2003	24,227	51,000,984	58.1	4893	6,058,383	140.3
2004	23,721	51,936,581	55.9	4815	6,247,820	137.1
2005	23,593	52,836,948	54.2	4822	6,441,264	132.5
2006	23,197	53,628,655	51.9	4693	6,621,700	124.8
2007	23,660	54,358,003	51.6	4905	6,786,059	127.5
2008	23,357	55,076,324	49.6	4585	6,952,690	114.1
2009	22,777	55,818,210	47.3	4793	7,117,230	114.7
2010	23,167	56,625,960	46.7	4853	7,300,035	111.8
2011	22,725	57,346,700	44.7	4656	7,454,519	102.3
2012	22,084	57,948,688	42.1	4594	7,597,131	97.1

observations—one for each year for each race. We would like to examine trends over time within each race group, so we include a term for year, a term for race, and a term for the interaction between race and year, allowing us to formally test whether the trend differs by race. The full model is:

$$\log(\text{Deaths}_i) = \log(\text{Population}_i) + \beta_0 + \beta_1 \text{Year}_i + \beta_2 \text{Race}_i + \beta_3 \text{Year}_i \times \text{Race}_i,$$

where $i = 1, \ldots, 46$ index observations, year denotes years since 1990, and race is a binary indicator (0 for white men and 1 for black men).

Table 5.5 shows the estimated relative risks (exponentiated regression coefficients) from three Poisson regression models. The first model omits the population exposure and the interaction term. The second model adds the exposure, and the third model adds the exposure and the interaction. The stark difference between the first two sets of results clearly demonstrates the critical role of the exposure in the analysis.

When we omit the exposure, the regression is modeling the counts of deaths each year. The number of deaths is much lower among black men than among white

Table 5.5 Three Poisson regression models fit to annual prostate cancer deaths

Model	Exposure	Interaction	Predictor	Relative risk	95% CI	P-value
1	No	No	Race = Black	0.20	(0.20, 0.20)	<0.001
1	No	No	Year	0.99	(0.99, 0.99)	<0.001
2	Yes	No	Race = Black	1.75	(1.74, 1.76)	<0.001
2	Yes	No	Year	0.97	(0.97, 0.97)	<0.001
3	Yes	Yes	Race = Black	1.93	(1.90, 1.95)	<0.001
3	Yes	Yes	Year	0.97	(0.97, 0.97)	<0.001
3	Yes	Yes	Race = Black × Year	0.99	(0.99, 0.99)	<0.001

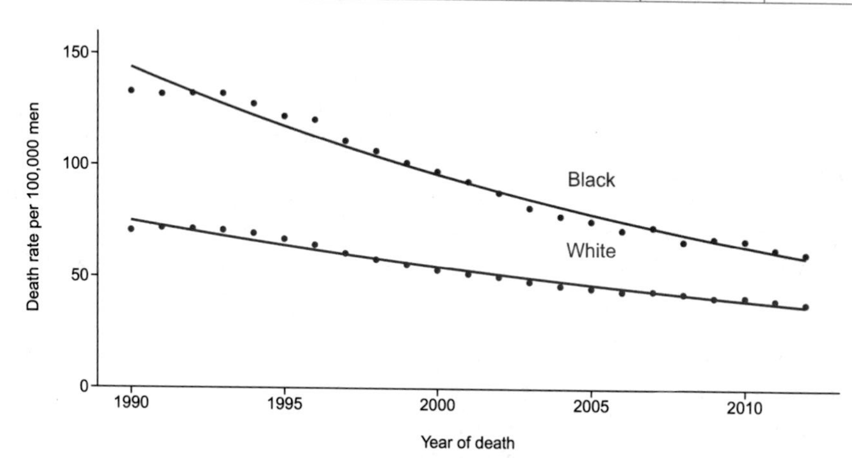

Fig. 5.3 Observed (dots) and fitted (solid lines) prostate cancer mortality rates from a Poisson regression model accounting for population size and interaction between race and year

men; the model estimates an 80% lower risk of prostate cancer death in black men relative to white men. But this estimate disregards the much smaller size of the black population.

When we include the exposure, the regression is modeling the rates of deaths each year. The model with the exposure shows that the annual death rate among blacks is almost double that among whites, which comports with historic observation in the United States. Without an interaction term, the model assumes a similar effect of year for black and white men and estimates a 3% decline in the death rate each year. In the model which allows for a different effect of year for black and white men, the model estimates a 3% annual decline for white men and a 4% annual decline for black men. The fitted faster decline for black men is statistically significant as evidenced by the p-value for the interaction term. Figure 5.3 illustrates this interaction model graphically.

We have seen how Poisson regression can be used to model numbers of events for individuals and numbers of persons experiencing an event in populations. The concept of exposure, which quantifies opportunity to record the event, is applicable in both settings. In the individual setting, the exposure might capture a time duration or spatial area over which subjects are at risk for the event. In the population setting, the exposure is the size of the eligible population. Analyses that include an offset term representing the exposure facilitate inferences about event rates (i.e., mean events per unit exposure) as opposed to analyses that do not include the offset, which provide inferences about event counts and do not standardize by the exposure.

5.6 Overdispersion, Negative Binomial, and Zero-Inflated Models

The main limitation of the Poisson regression model for count outcomes is its strong modeling assumptions. While the model accommodates a variance that increases with the mean, the rigid relationship between the mean and the variance is often not satisfied in practice.

Figure 5.4 shows the variance of the number of outpatient visits in the BHP example as a function of the mean. The means were calculated using the estimated coefficients from the model in Table 5.3, and the variances were calculated for groups of observations with similar estimated means. When the Poisson assumption holds, the variances should follow the $x = y$ line, where the mean and variance are equal. However, the variance in this example is clearly greater than the mean. The data are said to be *overdispersed*.

In practice, an overdispersed count outcome may have more observations that are zero or more observations that are large (or both) compared to what would be expected under a Poisson distribution. Thus, compared with a Poisson distribution,

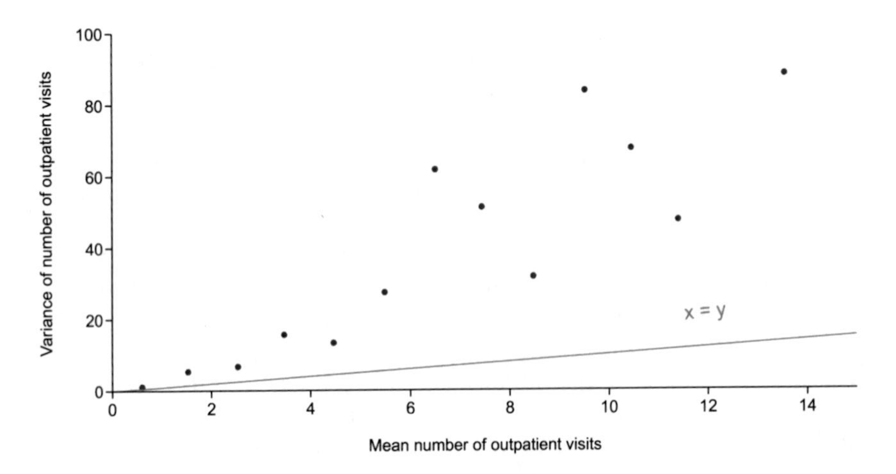

Fig. 5.4 Mean number of outpatient visits from the Poisson regression in Table 5.3 and variances among observations with similar predicted means (purple dots) and the expected relationship between the mean and variance if the Poisson assumption holds (green line)

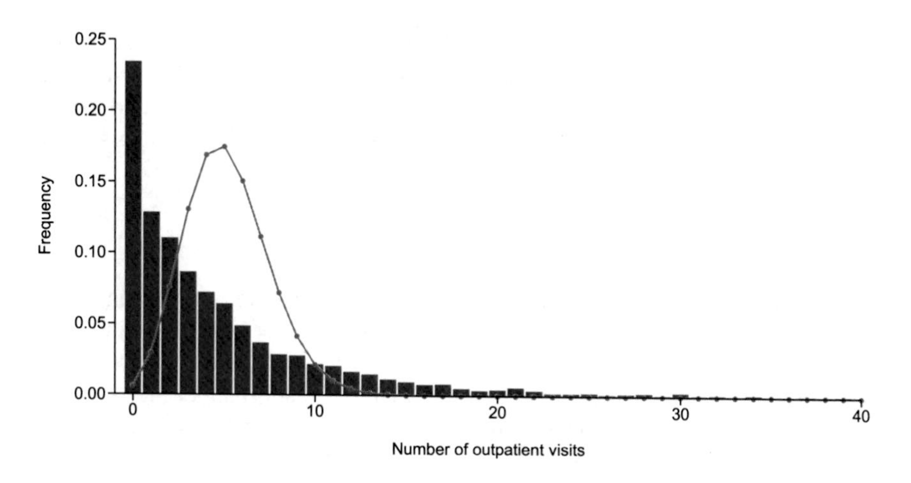

Fig. 5.5 Histogram of number of outpatient visits (gray bars), truncated at 40, in the Basic Health Plan and the Poisson probability density function with the same mean (red line and points)

the histogram showing the distribution of an overdispersed outcome may have a spike at zero and/or a longer right tail than a Poisson distribution with the same mean. As shown in Fig. 5.5, both of these features are evident in the BHP data.

Failing to account for overdispersion in count data models may lead to inaccurate inferences, such as hypothesis tests that are incorrectly sized and confidence intervals that do not achieve the assumed level of coverage.

5.6.1 Negative Binomial Regression

When count data are overdispersed, negative binomial regression is commonly used. A negative binomial regression has the same mean structure as a Poisson regression but adds an extra parameter to accommodate variance over and above the mean.

In Chap. 2, we showed that the negative binomial distribution can be thought of as an extended version of the Poisson distribution that explicitly allows each person to deviate from the common mean model in an individual-specific way. For example, individuals are heterogeneous with respect to their health care utilization, with some requiring a great deal of care and others requiring little or none. We might imagine that each individual has an underlying, unobserved level of health that predicts the intensity of health care utilization as captured by the count outcome. This would manifest in practice as different rates of utilization for different individuals, even if they share exactly the same predictor values. A person who has frequent outpatient visits in the current time period is more likely to have frequent visits in the next time period. Hence, due to between-patient heterogeneity, the assumption of independence of counts across different time intervals is violated.

How can we express this idea of individual heterogeneity in outpatient visits in the BHP example? Mathematically, we may consider each individual's count outcome Y_i to have a Poisson distribution with mean μ_i as in standard Poisson regression. But now, instead of μ_i being solely a function of the predictors X_i, we could write μ_i as:

$$\mu_i = r_i \gamma_i,$$

where γ_i depends linearly on the predictors X_i and r_i is a random, person-specific multiplier sometimes called a *random effect*. In this way, persons having the same predictor values share the same γ, but their expectations of the outcome differ according to the person-specific r multiplier. Higher r_i means that person i tends to have more frequent events and lower r_i means that person tends to have less frequent events.

It should be immediately apparent that including heterogeneity across individuals in this way will add variability to the outcome. A negative binomial distribution is a distribution for count data outcomes that captures this variability. Formally, the negative binomial results from imposing a specific distribution over the factors r_i. If the distribution is a gamma distribution with mean 1 and variance α, one can show that Y_i follows a negative binomial distribution with mean given by:

$$E(Y_i) = \gamma_i,$$

and variance given by:

$$\text{Var}(Y_i) = \gamma_i(1 + \alpha\gamma_i).$$

Using this framework to accommodate heterogeneity, a log-linear model for γ_i, namely:

$$\log(\gamma_i) = \beta_0 + \beta_1 X_{1i} + \cdots + \beta_k X_{ki},$$

leaves us with exactly the same log-linear model for $E(Y_i)$, with the same mean structure and interpretation, only now with a distribution that has greater variance than the mean. A higher value of α increases the variance relative to the Poisson distribution with the same mean as shown in Fig. 5.6. The overdispersion parameter α must be estimated as part of the model-fitting process. When $\alpha = 0$, there is no overdispersion, and this can be checked via a likelihood-ratio test or by using the Akaike Information Criterion (AIC) or Bayesian Information Criterion (BIC) to compare the negative binomial and Poisson models.

Table 5.6 shows the results of a negative binomial regression applied to the BHP data using the enrollment duration as the exposure offset. Comparison of the estimates from this model with the corresponding Poisson regression model (Table 5.3) shows that allowing for overdispersion has only a modest impact on the coefficient estimates but a more pronounced impact on the p-values associated

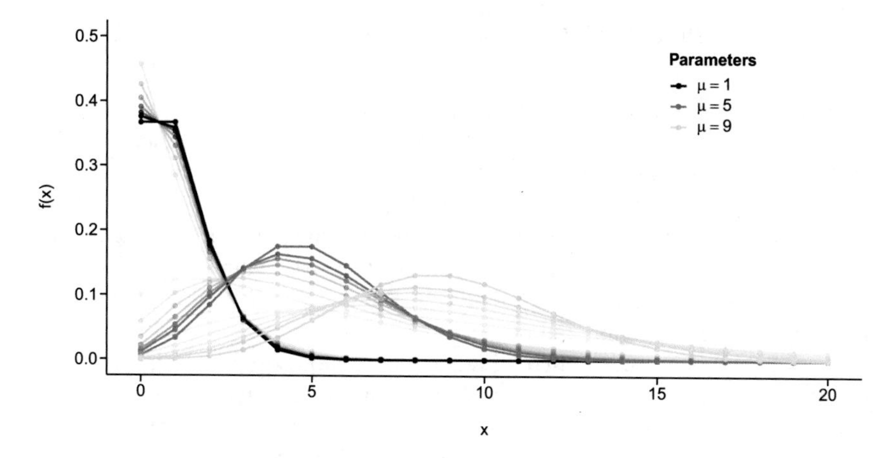

Fig. 5.6 Poisson probability density functions for different values of the mean μ (solid, opaque lines) and negative binomial density functions with the same mean and different values of the dispersion parameter α (semi-transparent lines)

Table 5.6 Fitted negative binomial regression of outpatient visits in the Basic Health Plan including the exposure variable adjusted for age, sex, race, and number of chronic conditions. Estimated risks are relative to Spokane HMO

Provider	Coefficient	Relative risk	95% CI	P-value
Spokane IPA	0.01	1.01	(0.90, 1.13)	> 0.9
Pierce	0.09	1.10	(1.01, 1.19)	0.03
Clallam	−0.04	0.96	(0.86, 1.07)	0.5

Table 5.7 AIC and BIC for standard and zero-inflated Poisson and negative binomial models fit to outpatient visits in the Basic Health Plan

Model	Exposure	AIC	BIC
Poisson	No	28,344	28,411
Poisson	Yes	22,938	23,005
Negative binomial	Yes	16,425	16,498
Zero-inflated Poisson	Yes	21,066	21,200
Zero-inflated negative binomial	Yes	16,392	16,532

with various hypothesis tests. Both the formal test for $\alpha = 0$ and the AIC and BIC, shown in Table 5.7, indicate that the negative binomial model is preferred. This is not unexpected given the relative magnitudes of the means and variances in Table 5.1.

5.6.2 Zero-Inflated Count Data Regression

Zero-inflated count data models accommodate settings where the number of observations with an outcome of zero exceeds what would be expected under Poisson or negative binomial models. This might occur in health care utilization settings, for example, when we study counts of outpatient visits.

Excess zeros in the outcome variable can be caused by a variety of factors. One factor, as noted above, is overdispersion—we may be dealing with an outcome variable that varies more than is captured by the Poisson distribution assumed for the analysis. Another factor could be structural.

A structural zero occurs when an individual cannot experience the event being counted. In the case of outpatient visits, for example, an individual without access to the health care system who cannot see a doctor, and who therefore has zero outpatient visits, would generate a structural zero. If we had an indicator of health care access, we could partition our sample into those who could and those who could not access the system. We might model the access indicator using a binary outcome model (e.g., logistic regression) and the number of visits among those with access using a count data model (e.g., Poisson regression). This type of two-part modeling approach is discussed in Chap. 6.

What if we do not have an indicator of health care access in the data? Zero-inflated count data models are designed for this setting.

A zero-inflated count data distribution reflects a mixture of two populations: one in which counts follow a distribution such as a Poisson or negative binomial distribution and another in which all observations are zero. If an observed outcome is non-zero, then we know that it was generated by the first population; if it is zero, we can never know definitively whether it came from the first or the second population. However, we can still estimate the probability p that it comes from the first population by comparing the observed fraction of outcomes that are zero with the fraction that would be expected under the specified distribution for the counts. Both the count data distribution and the probability of belonging to it, p, can be modeled using predictors. Thus, when specifying a zero-inflated model, we specify two regression models: one for the count outcomes and one for the excess zeros.

In principle, the predictors for the two components of zero-inflated models can be the same or different; in practice, the coefficient estimates, particularly for the excess zero component, must be interpreted with caution. These estimates are not based on observed indicators; instead, they are derived to best fit the observed data given the specified count data model. In a sense, the excess-zero model estimation serves to “mop up” any excess in the number of zero outcomes relative to what would be expected under the specified count data model fit to the observed data. As we have already seen, if the count data model is negative binomial, there is a built-in expectation that the distribution will include a greater fraction of zeros than if the count data model is Poisson. Therefore, the estimated zero-inflated model could be very different if the distribution for the count outcome is specified to be negative binomial than if the distribution for the count outcome is specified to be Poisson.

Table 5.8 Fitted zero-inflated Poisson regression of outpatient visits in the Basic Health Plan including the exposure variable adjusted for age, sex, race, and number of chronic conditions. Estimated risks are relative to Spokane HMO

Component	Provider	Relative risk	95% CI	P-value
Zero model	Spokane IPA	1.16	(0.80, 1.69)	0.4
Count model	Spokane IPA	1.04	(0.99, 1.10)	0.12
Zero model	Pierce	1.05	(0.79, 1.40)	0.7
Count model	Pierce	1.13	(1.09, 1.17)	<0.001
Zero model	Clallam	1.15	(0.80, 1.65)	0.5
Count model	Clallam	0.97	(0.92, 1.03)	0.3

Table 5.9 Fitted zero-inflated negative binomial regression of outpatient visits in the Basic Health Plan including the exposure variable adjusted for age, sex, race, and number of chronic conditions. Estimated risks are relative to Spokane HMO

Component	Provider	Relative risk	95% CI	P-value
Zero model	Spokane IPA	0.95	(0.34, 2.64)	>0.9
Count model	Spokane IPA	1.00	(0.89, 1.12)	>0.9
Zero model	Pierce	1.16	(0.63, 2.12)	0.6
Count model	Pierce	1.11	(1.02, 1.20)	0.02
Zero model	Clallam	1.12	(0.48, 2.59)	0.8
Count model	Clallam	0.96	(0.86, 1.08)	0.5

Tables 5.8 and 5.9 shows the results of fitting two zero-inflated models to outpatient visits in the BHP example. The first table specifies a Poisson model for the count data outcome, and the second table specifies a negative binomial model. Both tables give the exponentiated coefficient estimates, which are interpretable as relative risks for the number of outpatient visits and as relative odds for the probability of an excess zero. The only statistically significant effects are for the count data model; the mean number of outpatient visits is estimated to be 13% higher and 11% higher for the Pierce provider than the reference provider (Spokane HMO) under the Poisson and negative binomial models, respectively. The probability of having excess zeros does not differ across providers (all p-values 0.4 or greater). Thus, the fitted models seem to suggest that the distribution of outpatient visits does not have a structural zero component that differs across providers. This is consistent with the fact that all participants had access to health care in the BHP program regardless of their provider.

We can determine whether the zero-inflated model is preferred to a pure count model by evaluating the change in AIC and BIC. A commonly cited test for the same purpose, the Vuong test [7], has been shown to be not technically correct and capable of producing biased results [8]. Table 5.7 shows the AIC and BIC results for the Poisson and negative binomial models and their zero-inflated versions fit to the BHP data. The zero-inflated versions provide relatively modest improvement over the non-inflated models (except the BIC for a negative binomial count model).

5.7 Generalized Linear Models

We conclude this chapter by introducing the family of generalized linear models (GLMs), first defined and characterized by Nelder and Wedderburn [9]. The family of GLMs provides a unifying framework that includes linear and logistic regression as well as the (non-zero-inflated) Poisson and negative binomial count data regression models.

A GLM is specified by defining three features:

1. A *distribution* of Y given μ that is a member of the so-called *exponential family* of distributions. This family includes the normal, binomial, Poisson, gamma, and negative binomial distributions.
2. A *linear predictor* $\beta_0 + \beta_1 X_{1i} + \cdots + \beta_k X_{ki}$ that defines the joint effect of the predictors.
3. A *link function*, $g(\cdot)$, that links between the mean (or *expected value*) of the outcome $\mu = E(Y)$ and the linear predictor:

$$g(\mu) = \beta_0 + \beta_1 X_{1i} + \cdots + \beta_k X_{ki}.$$

   We usually match the range of the link function to the range of μ. Thus, for example, if μ ranges between zero and one, as is the case with binary outcomes, then we might use the logit function for g, which maps this interval to the real line.

Once these three features are specified, an expression for the implied distribution can be generated. Every GLM's distributional specification follows the same formula. Examples include:

- A normal distribution with an identity link for linear regression
- A binomial distribution with a logit link for logistic regression
- A Poisson distribution with a log link for Poisson regression.

The variance of the model is usually implied by the distribution of Y, and, in most cases, it is a function of the mean μ, except for the normal distribution, in which case the link function is specified to be the identify function.

The value of having a unifying family of models is that statistical methods or properties that are based on the structure of the members of the family can be broadly applied to all of the members of the family. Thus, for example, a single algorithm, iteratively reweighted least squares, was developed by Nelder and Wedderburn [9] for maximum likelihood estimation for all GLMs. Similarly, generalized estimating equations, a method used to estimate GLMs when observations are correlated, leverages the general formula for the score equation (i.e., the derivative of the log likelihood) of a GLM. In Chap. 6, the use of GLM is exploited for continuous outcomes with right-skewed distributions.

In statistical software packages, GLMs can typically be fit either by a call to a specific type of regression function (e.g., logistic or Poisson) or by a call to a GLM function that takes as input parameters the distribution and link function specifications. Not all distribution and link function combinations are compatible. For example, a logit link will generally not be applicable to real-valued data from a normal distribution.

GLMs can be compared using likelihood-based statistics, including likelihood ratio tests (for nested models) and the AIC and BIC for nested and non-nested models. The *deviance*, a term generally reserved for use with GLMs, is a goodness-of-fit statistic for a given model that essentially measures the difference between the maximum log likelihood for that model and the log likelihood obtained when replacing each μ_i by its corresponding Y_i. Thus, the deviance takes the difference between the log likelihoods of the estimated model and the "fullest" model given the observed data. A lower deviance generally indicates a preferred model, but any performance improvements must be considered in the context of the additional parameters required to improve the fit of the model.

In principle, there are many combinations of distributions and link functions that might be applied to analyze health utilization outcomes. However, only a few GLMs are used in practice. Beyond the well-known and frequently applied models listed above, a gamma distribution with a log link function has become popular for analyzing skewed health care costs (see Chap. 6). A binomial distribution with a log link is sometimes used to produce binary regression results that are interpretable as relative risks rather than relative odds, but standard estimation algorithms can fail to converge in some cases because the log link is not always compatible with the constraint that the mean of a binomial distribution must lie between 0 and 1. This can be addressed using a modified estimation approach [10, 11] or via marginal effect estimation.

All GLMs with non-linear link functions g share the feature that coefficient estimates (βs) are interpretable in terms of how they affect $g(\mu)$ rather than how they affect the mean μ itself. Transforming the coefficient estimates into meaningful quantities (i.e., additive or multiplicative effects on the mean μ) must be explicitly addressed as part of the analysis. We have already encountered this problem in logistic regression, where a regression coefficient β is interpretable as the change in logit(μ) corresponding to a one-unit change in the corresponding predictor X. The technique of recycled predictions, introduced in this setting, to obtain marginal effect estimates of a change in X on μ is applicable across GLMs with non-linear link functions. Ultimately, the GLM family provides not only a unifying framework for an array of models; it also encompasses a suite of methods that apply across the entire family and facilitate analysis of a broad array of health outcomes.

5.8 Software and Data

R code to download data and to carry out the examples in this book is available at the GitHub page https://roman-gulati.github.io/statistics-for-health-data-science/. Data on outpatient visits from the Basic Health Plan of Washington State and prostate cancer mortality from the Surveillance, Epidemiology, and End Results program are also provided. In addition to the R packages cited in Chap. 1, this chapter also used the `MASS` [12], `lmtest` [13], `pscl` [14], and `tableone` [15] packages.

References

1. McCullagh, P., Nelder, J.A.: Generalized Linear Models. Chapman & Hall/CRC, London (1989)
2. Martin, D.P., Diehr, P., Cheadle, A., Madden, C.W., Patrick, D.L., Skillman, S.M.: Health care utilization for the "newly insured": Results from the Washington Basic Health Plan. Inquiry **34**, 129–142 (1997)
3. National Cancer Institute: Surveillance, Epidemiology, and End Results, http://seer.cancer.gov/registries/. Accessed 12 February 2020
4. Siegel, R.L., Miller, K.D., Jemal, A.: Cancer statistics, 2020. CA Cancer J. Clin. **70**, 7–30 (2020). https://doi.org/10.3322/caac.21590
5. Gross, C.P., Andersen, M.S., Krumholz, H.M., McAvay, G.J., Proctor, D., Tinetti, M.E.: Relation between Medicare screening reimbursement and stage at diagnosis for older patients with colon cancer. J. Am. Med. Assoc. **296**, 2815–2822 (2006). https://doi.org/10.1001/jama.296.23.2815
6. Holford, T.R., Cronin, K.A., Mariotto, A.B., Feuer, E.J.: Changing patterns in breast cancer incidence trends. J. Natl. Cancer Inst. Monogr. **36**, 19–25 (2006). https://doi.org/10.1093/jncimonographs/lgj016
7. Vuong, Q.H.: Likelihood ratio tests for model selection and non-nested hypotheses. Econometrica **57**, 307–333 (1989)
8. Wilson, P.: The misuse of the Vuong test for non-nested models to test for zero-inflation. Econ. Lett. **127**, 51–53 (2015). https://doi.org/10.1016/j.econlet.2014.12.029
9. Nelder, J., Wedderburn, R.: Generalized linear models. J. R. Stat. Soc. Ser. A **135**, 370–384 (1972). https://doi.org/10.2307/2344614
10. Marschner, I.C., Gillett, A.C.: Relative risk regression: reliable and flexible methods for log-binomial models. Biostatistics **13**, 179–192 (2012)
11. Donoghoe, M.W., Marschner, I.C.: Flexible regression models for rate differences, risk differences and relative risks. Int. J. Biostat. **11**, 91–108 (2015)
12. Venables, W.N., Ripley, B.D.: Modern Applied Statistics with S, 4th edn. Springer, New York (2002). http://www.stats.ox.ac.uk/pub/MASS4. ISBN 0-387-95457-0
13. Zeileis, A., Kleiber, C., Jackman, S.: Regression models for count data in R. J. Stat. Softw. **27**(8) (2008). http://www.jstatsoft.org/v27/i08/
14. Jackman, S.: pscl: Classes and Methods for R Developed in the Political Science Computational Laboratory. United States Studies Centre, University of Sydney, Sydney, New South Wales, Australia (2020). https://github.com/atahk/pscl/. R package version 1.5.5
15. Yoshida, K.: tableone: Create 'Table 1' to Describe Baseline Characteristics (2020). https://github.com/kaz-yos/tableone. R package version 0.11.1

Chapter 6
Health Care Costs

Abstract This chapter introduces specialized regression methods for health cost outcomes. After considering what we mean by health care expenditures, we introduce several regression models for right-skewed expenditure outcomes. Standard linear regression modeling of the logarithm of the outcome is a classical solution to the problem of right-skewed outcome data. We introduce the lognormal distribution, which this approach implicitly assumes, and discuss the problem of retransforming the coefficient estimates back to the original cost metric. To avoid retransformation issues, we consider a gamma generalized linear model that accommodates the right-skewed nature of the outcome without needing to transform it. The lognormal and gamma models can only model positive expenditures, but when individuals do not use the health care system, and consequently do not incur any expenditures over the observation interval, the distribution of health care costs includes a mass at zero. To address this, we introduce the two-part model, which models separately the probability of incurring expenditures and the mean expenditures incurred. A final step combines the two parts of the model to produce marginal estimates of covariate effects. We end with a discussion of other analytic approaches for health expenditure outcomes, including models for median expenditures.

6.1 Defining and Measuring Health Care Costs

What is a health care cost? It turns out that this simple question is surprisingly difficult to answer. There are different perspectives involved, and the cost of care means different things—and potentially different amounts—under each [1]. To patients, the cost is the amount they pay out of pocket for care in the form of insurance deductibles, co-payments, or non-covered services. To payers, it is the amount reimbursed to providers for services rendered. To providers, it is the expenses incurred to deliver the relevant services; over the long run, these expenses must cover not only the costs of producing the services themselves but also the supporting costs. A quote from Brownlee et al. [2] about the provider costs of giving a patient a CT scan is instructive: "a hospital has to have purchased a scanner. It must also pay a technologist to perform the scan and a radiologist to read it—to

R. Etzioni et al., *Statistics for Health Data Science*, Springer Texts in Statistics,
https://doi.org/10.1007/978-3-030-59889-1_6

say nothing of paying for the hospital building itself, chairs in the waiting room, a receptionist at the information desk, and the parking lot outside, all of which are components of the cost of a scan."

When describing health care costs, various terms may be used. Arora et al. [1] discusses charges, payments, and expenditures. The charges on a medical bill or claim do not reflect any of the aforementioned perspectives. Rather, they are an attempt to initiate negotiation beginning with a relatively high bar, knowing that the payer will ultimately pay a lower amount. Payments, the amounts reimbursed, are likely closer to actual health care costs than charges, but they don't include out-of-pocket expenses. And payments may vary depending on the insurer and the setting (e.g., hospital versus outpatient). Ultimately, there is no absolute concept of health care costs. For a given patient in a given health care setting and with a given payer, the closest approximation to a health care cost may be total expenditures associated with the service. This quantity is the sum of the insurance payment, the out-of-pocket amount, and any expenses associated with the health plan (e.g., insurance premium, deductible, and co-payment if not included in the out-of-pocket amount). This expenditure-centric concept will constitute our definition of health care costs in this chapter.

6.2 MEPS Data on Health Care Utilization and Costs

The Medical Expenditure Panel Survey (MEPS) [3] provides a rich resource for studying health care utilization and expenditures in the United States. MEPS has been fielded since 1996 and is designed to provide timely information about the nation's changing health care system. A new cohort is enrolled each year and interviewed five times over a period of two years. Thus, the survey has a rolling panel design, with participants in a given year consisting of both those enrolled that year and those enrolled in the prior year. The MEPS database includes data on participant socio-demographics, health behaviors, existing conditions, and access to care. In addition to surveying participants about their encounters with the health care system, MEPS also requests detailed information about medical expenses, charges, and payments—both covered and out-of-pocket—for these services. The Medical Provider Component of MEPS reports responses from a sample of providers to corroborate information submitted and impute missing data. The MEPS data aggregate health care costs into separate expenditure variables for inpatient, outpatient, and office-based care, prescription medications, and out-of-pocket expenditures. Although MEPS follows a complex survey design including stratification, clustering, and weighting, these topics are postponed to Chap. 9; we do not use the survey design variables to produce the results in this chapter.

The unique compilation of health status, health behavior, and health expenditure variables in MEPS, in addition to its public accessibility, has made it a go-to resource for studying the health expenditures associated with a variety of conditions,

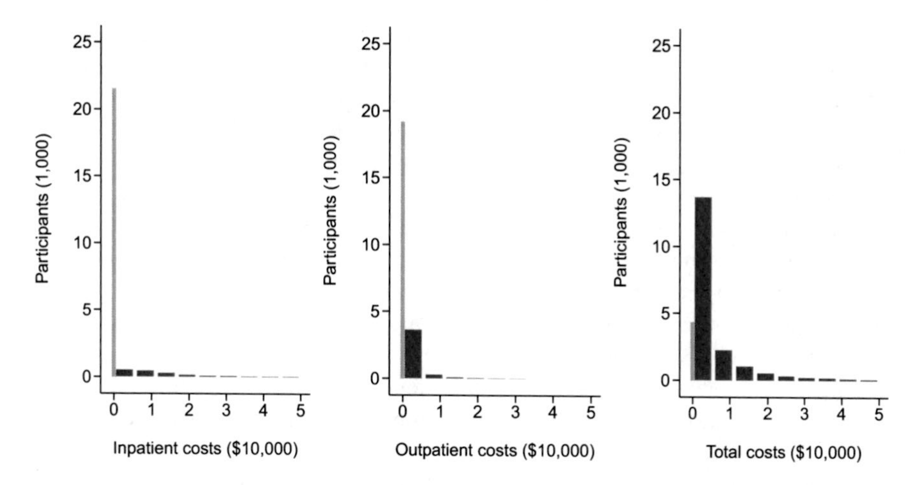

Fig. 6.1 Histograms of inpatient, outpatient, and total medical expenditures in MEPS 2017 data for participants age 18 years or older. The orange bars show numbers of participants with zero costs. All costs were truncated at $50,000

Table 6.1 Summary statistics of inpatient, outpatient, and total medical expenditures in MEPS 2017 data for participants age 18 years or older. Statistics are reported separately for all participants and for participants with non-zero medical expenditures

Group	Statistic	Inpatient	Outpatient	Total
Overall	No. of participants	23,373	23,373	23,373
Overall	Mean costs	$1388	$523	$5927
Overall	Median costs	$0	$0	$1189
Overall	Percent with zero costs	92%	82%	19%
Non-zero costs	No. of participants	1810	4156	19,022
Non-zero costs	Mean costs	$17,925	$2941	$7283
Non-zero costs	Median costs	$9857	$710	$2026

including chronic pain [4], obesity [5, 6], and hypertension [7]. MEPS has also been used to study changes in medical expenditures in relation to health policies [8].

Figure 6.1 displays a set of histograms showing the distribution of annual overall costs and different components of costs for adults in the MEPS 2017 dataset. All these expenditure distributions are extremely right skewed. In the case of total costs, for example, 5% of respondents account for more than 50% of the expenditures. All histograms also show a large number of participants with zero expenditures (orange bars). Table 6.1 gives the fraction of individuals with zero expenditures and the mean and median expenditures overall and for participants with non-zero expenditures. 81% of MEPS respondents had some expenditures, but only 8% had inpatient expenditures and only 18% had outpatient expenditures in 2017.

In practice, the underlying scientific question of interest determines whether it is more appropriate to summarize overall costs with a single number or to identify the proportion with zero costs and to summarize costs only among persons with non-zero costs. For example, if evaluating efforts to expand access in underserved populations, it may be more useful to tease apart changes in the proportion with zero costs versus changes in costs among persons who already have access to health care. Similarly, the underlying scientific question determines whether it is more appropriate to use the mean or the median (or another statistic) to summarize a skewed distribution.

Given the heterogeneity of health care expenditures, the predictors and correlates of these expenditures are of great interest. But the extremely non-normal nature of cost outcomes means that standard linear regression analyses may not be appropriate for inference. In this chapter, we explore models and methods that have been developed expressly for these types of outcomes. We begin by examining methods for highly skewed outcomes with a focus on analyses of mean expenditures.

As an illustrative analysis, we will examine the relationship between a prior diagnosis of diabetes and total medical expenditures. Diabetes has long been recognized as an urgent and growing health problem in the United States. According to the Centers for Disease Control and Prevention [9], the prevalence of diabetes among US adults age 18 or older is 13%; among those over 65, the prevalence doubles to 27%. Individuals with diabetes have a host of comorbidities and potential complications: 89% are overweight or obese, 68% have high blood pressure, and 44% have high cholesterol. Complications include cardiovascular disease and nerve damage leading to foot ulcers, retinopathies, and kidney damage. Managing diabetes involves managing the condition as well as any of these complications; it has been documented [10] that direct medical costs following a diabetes diagnosis are on average 2.3 times those in the absence of diabetes. In this chapter, we study the incremental costs associated with diabetes among adult respondents to the MEPS 2017. We control for age, sex, and race/ethnicity but not for BMI or other comorbidities. Thus, our estimates of incremental cost include those attributable to diabetes as well as to other comorbidities that tend to be present in diabetes cases.

6.3 Log Cost Models and the Lognormal Distribution

A classical approach for regression modeling of a right-skewed outcome on the positive real line is to use standard linear regression with the log-transformed outcome, $\log(Y)$. The motivation here is that if the outcome is highly skewed, the log transformation will make it normal—or at least normal enough that linear regression is valid.

Why does this work? The answer has to do with the log transformation and its inverse, the exponential transformation. The log transformation is a compressive function; applied to a set of positive numbers, it shrinks those at the higher end of the range more than those at the lower end. The base 10 log of 1000, written $\log_{10}(1000)$, is 3; $\log_{10}(100)$ is 2, $\log_{10}(10)$ is 1, and $\log_{10}(1)$ is 0. So the $\log_{10}$ transformation turns a range from 1 to 1000 into a range from 0 to 3. Consequently, the log transformation is a natural choice to effectively "pull in" high Y values that appear in the upper tail of a right-skewed distribution, narrowing its range. The same is true for log transformations using other bases, such as the natural logarithm (often written simply "log") which has base $e \approx 2.7$. The inverse of the natural logarithm, the exponential transformation (often written "exp"), is a magnifying function; applied to a set of numbers, it stretches those at the higher end of the range more than those at the lower end. Here, as in other chapters of this book, we use the natural basis whenever we apply a logarithmic or exponential transformation.

When we take the log of Y and apply standard linear regression, we are often making an implicit assumption, namely, that $\log(Y)$ is normally distributed. Formally, we write:

$$\log(Y) \sim N(\mu, \sigma^2).$$

In the case where Y is costs, $\log(Y)$ is the log of costs, μ is the mean of log costs, and σ^2 is the variance of log costs. In the regression setting with covariates $X_1, \ldots,$ X_k, the model is:

$$\log(Y \mid X_1, \ldots, X_k) \sim N(\beta_0 + \beta_1 X_1 + \cdots + \beta_k X_k, \sigma^2),$$

where β_0, β_1, …, β_k are the regression coefficients that represent an intercept and the effects of a change in the corresponding covariate on the mean of $\log(Y)$.

Given our familiarity with the normal distribution and standard linear regression (see Chap. 3), we know how to estimate μ or the βs. The βs quantify the association between the covariates X and the mean of $\log(Y)$. However, health care costs are not easily understood in log dollars; ideally we would like estimates of the effects of covariates on the mean of Y. In short, when our model is for $E[\log(Y)] = \mu$, then what is $E(Y)$? As we pointed out in Chap. 2, it turns out that $E(Y)$ is not simply $\exp(\mu)$, the inverse transformation of μ. This happens because when we log or exponentiate a random variable, we change its entire distribution. We demonstrate this using a simple example.

The left panel of Fig. 6.2 shows two normal distributions with mean zero and variances 1 and 4. These can be thought of as representing distributions of $\log(Y)$ for two different Ys, say inpatient and outpatient expenditures measured in log dollars. Let's call these random variables Z_1 and Z_2. Theoretically, both Z_1 and Z_2 can take values across the entire real line, but most of the values of Z_1 (the purple curve) fall within a much narrower range than the values of Z_2 (the green curve). Similarly, a given probability (say 20%) in the upper tail covers a set of values that is less extreme for Z_1 than Z_2.

When we exponentiate Z_1 and Z_2, we generate the variables $Y_1 = \exp(Z_1)$ and $Y_2 = \exp(Z_2)$ that are now measured in dollars. The distributions shift from being on the entire real line to being on the non-negative real line. And the probability associated with any interval on the original scale becomes associated with the exponentiated values of that interval. Consequently, the same probability (say 20%) in the upper tail shifts from covering the extreme values of Z_1 and Z_2 to covering the corresponding extreme values of $\exp(Z_1)$ and $\exp(Z_2)$.

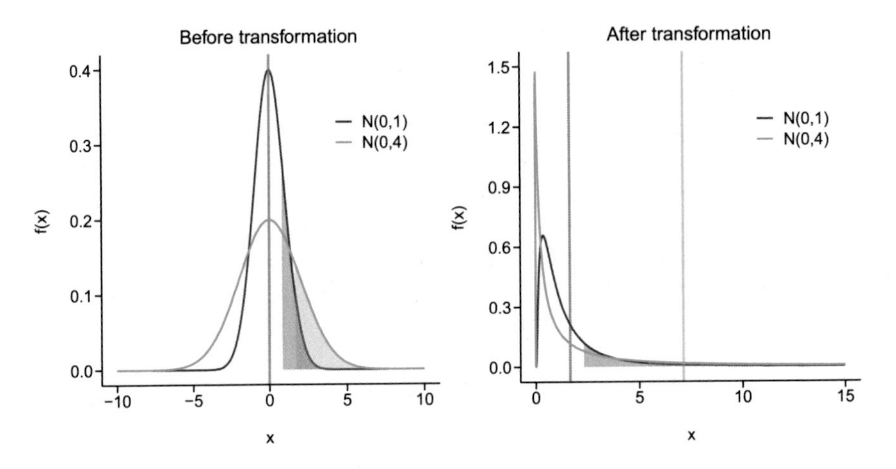

Fig. 6.2 Densities of two normal distributions with the same mean and different variances before (left) and after (right) exponential transformation. Shaded areas show 20% probability in the upper tail of each distribution. Vertical lines show the mean of each distribution

The right panel of Fig. 6.2 shows the distributions of Y_1 and Y_2, which are both right skewed. But the distribution of Y_2 is more right skewed than that of Y_1, so it is reasonable to guess that Y_2 has a higher mean than Y_1 (and indeed it has). We began with two random variables with the same mean and different variances. When we exponentiated them, we ended up with two random variables with different means and different variances.

In general, when we exponentiate a normal random variable, the result has a lognormal distribution. The mean of the lognormal random variable depends not only on the mean of the original random variable but also on its variance. Formally, when $E[\log(Y)] = \mu$ and $\text{Var}[\log(Y)] = \sigma^2$, then:

$$E(Y) = \exp\left(\mu + \frac{1}{2}\sigma^2\right) = \exp(\mu) \times \exp\left(\frac{1}{2}\sigma^2\right). \tag{6.1}$$

The mean of Y is the exponentiated mean of $\log(Y)$ multiplied by a term that depends on the variance. This multiplicative term is always larger than 1, and it increases with the variance of the normally distributed $\log(Y)$. As a consequence, when we fit a standard linear regression to log costs and we want to present results about effects of covariates in terms of dollars (not log dollars), we have to account for the log scale variance.

We first explore how this works in the setting of a single binary covariate X. Let $\log(Y)$ be the log of total expenditures among individuals with non-zero expenditures in the MEPS 2017 data, and consider the association between total expenditures and a prior diabetes diagnosis, where $X = 0$ indicates no prior diagnosis and $X = 1$ indicates a prior diagnosis. Suppose we fit a standard linear regression model to the log of expenditures, namely:

Table 6.2 Fitted linear regression of the log of positive total medical expenditures in MEPS 2017 for participants age 18 years or older

Predictor	Coefficient	SE	*P*-value
Intercept	7.386	0.013	< 0.001
Diabetes = yes	1.230	0.035	< 0.001

$$\log(Y) = \beta_0 + \beta_1 X + \epsilon,$$

where ϵ follows a normal distribution with mean zero and variance σ^2. This model implies that the mean of log expenditures increases by β_1 when X changes from 0 to 1. Further, σ^2 is the residual variance of $\log(Y)$, i.e., the variance of the log of expenditures not explained by a prior diabetes diagnosis.

Table 6.2 gives the results of this regression. (For simplicity, here and in the remainder of this chapter, 303 out of 23,373 persons with missing data on prior diabetes diagnosis were omitted.) In the table, the coefficient of the diabetes indicator is 1.23, telling us that the average log expenditures for participants with a prior diabetes diagnosis are 1.23 higher than the average log expenditures for participants without a prior diagnosis.

To obtain the implications of this model for the average medical expenditures, we can use Eq. (6.1). When our model is $\log(Y \mid X) \sim N(\beta_0 + \beta_1 X, \sigma^2)$, then:

$$E(Y \mid X) = \exp\left(\beta_0 + \beta_1 X + \frac{1}{2}\sigma^2\right) = \exp(\beta_0) \times \exp(\beta_1 X) \times \exp\left(\frac{1}{2}\sigma^2\right). \tag{6.2}$$

Thus, when we back-transform from the regression model scale to the original dollar scale, we have to account for the residual variance, σ^2. However, if this variance is the same for subjects with ($X = 1$) and without ($X = 0$) a prior diabetes diagnosis, we can show that:

$$\frac{E(Y \mid X = 1)}{E(Y \mid X = 0)} = \exp(\beta_1)$$

since the terms in Eq. (6.2) with the intercept and with the residual variance cancel. In this case, we would obtain the multiplicative effect of X on $E(Y)$ as $\exp(1.23) = 3.42$. Thus, we would infer that the average medical expenditures for participants with a prior diabetes diagnosis (who have positive expenditures) are 3.42 times the average medical expenditures for participants without a prior diagnosis.

If the residual variance is not the same across values of X, then we say that the data are *heteroskedastic*, and this affects how we estimate the effect of X on $E(Y)$ [11]. Let us write σ_0^2 and σ_1^2 for the residual variances of $\log(Y)$ when $X = 0$ and $X = 1$. Then, writing a separate version of Eq. (6.2) for each level of X, we obtain the effect of a prior diabetes diagnosis as:

$$\frac{E(Y \mid X=1)}{E(Y \mid X=0)} = \exp\left[\beta_1 + \frac{1}{2}\left(\sigma_1^2 - \sigma_0^2\right)\right]. \tag{6.3}$$

In the regression model summarized in Table 6.2, the residual variance for patients without a prior diabetes diagnosis is 2.93 (σ_0^2) and for those with a prior diagnosis is 2.46 (σ_1^2). Entering these values in Eq. (6.3), we obtain the multiplicative effect of a prior diabetes diagnosis on average medical expenditures as $\exp[1.23+0.5\times(2.46-2.93)] = 2.70$ among participants with any medical expenditures. Thus, taking the different residual variances into account, we would estimate that the average medical expenditures for participants with a prior diabetes diagnosis are 2.70 times the average medical expenditures for participants without a prior diagnosis.

Often, the variance increases with the mean, so if $\beta_1 > 0$, we expect $\sigma_1 > \sigma_0$ and $\exp(\beta_1)$ will underestimate the true effect. However, the variance and the mean may show different directions, and a negative effect may be associated with a positive β_1 coefficient. This is indeed the case in our example.

Because heteroskedasticity can sometimes create substantial bias in the estimates of covariate effects [11], it must be addressed in any analysis that retransforms results from a regression for log-transformed outcomes back to the original outcome scale. Tests for heteroskedasticity can be performed to determine whether this is likely to be a problem or not. One of the most well-known tests is the Breusch–Pagan test [12].

The null hypothesis for the Breusch–Pagan test is that the variance of the residuals from the regression model does not depend on the covariates in that regression model. To understand how this test works, we first need to remind ourselves how variance is defined and calculated.

The variance of a variable Z is just the average squared difference between the values of Z and its mean. Mathematically, this is written as $E\{[Z - E(Z)]^2\}$. In the case where Z represents the residual from a linear regression, the mean of Z is always zero, and the variance of the residuals from a standard linear regression is therefore just the mean of the squared residuals from that model, $\text{Var}(Z) = E(Z^2)$. Thus, to test whether the variance of the residuals depends on the covariates, the Breusch–Pagan test simply tests whether the mean of the squared residuals depends on the covariates. So, the Breusch–Pagan test effectively regresses the squared residuals from the fitted regression on the covariates and calculates a χ^2 goodness-of-fit statistic for a null hypothesis that there is no dependence on the covariates. When the goodness-of-fit statistic is large and dependence is indicated, the null hypothesis is rejected, and the analysis must account for heteroskedasticity in the retransformation step. Conversely, when the Breusch–Pagan test fails to reject the null hypothesis, the analysis usually proceeds as in the homoskedastic setting. We note however that, as discussed in Chap. 2, failing to reject a null hypothesis does not actually permit us to infer that it is true.

In the MEPS diabetes analysis, the Breusch–Pagan test is highly significant for this simple example and when we adjust for age, sex, and race/ethnicity (both p-values < 0.001). Because these adjustments themselves are highly significant and likely appropriate, we would report that the average medical expenditures among participants with a prior diabetes diagnosis were approximately 2.23 (the adjusted and heteroskedasticity-corrected estimate) times the average medical expenditures among participants without a prior diagnosis.

Dealing with heteroskedasticity across covariate categories may be manageable in the case of a single binary covariate, but it can become tedious and even prohibitive when there are multiple covariates of interest. Thus, contemporary models of average health care costs tend to use a different approach.

6.4 Gamma Models for Right-Skewed Cost Outcomes

The log cost model has traditionally been a staple for estimating the mean of right-skewed costs, but the potential for heteroskedasticity and the resulting retransformation issues limit its practical application. Ideally, one would model a cost outcome directly, in a way that avoids logging the costs. This would call for a regression modeling framework that accommodates a skewed distribution. The model should ideally allow for the variance to increase with the mean, as might be expected for health cost outcomes. And the effects of covariates on the outcome should be readily interpretable.

The gamma generalized linear model (GLM) with a log link satisfies all these requirements. The gamma distribution is a flexible distribution on the positive real line. It is specified by two parameters: α and β. The mean is α/β, and the variance is α/β^2, so the variance depends on the mean. Figure 6.3 reproduces a figure from Chap. 2 and shows some of the shapes that can be accommodated by the gamma distribution.

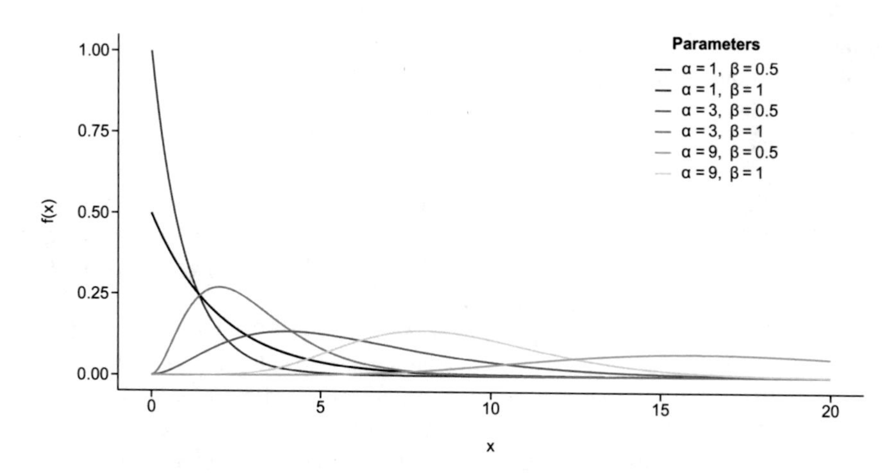

Fig. 6.3 Gamma density for different values of α and β

The "log link" means that the model relates the log of the mean to the linear predictor as follows:

$$\log[E(Y)] = \beta_0 + \beta_1 X_1 + \cdots + \beta_k X_k,$$

or equivalently:

$$E(Y) = \exp(\beta_0 + \beta_1 X_1 + \cdots + \beta_k X_k) = \exp(\beta_0) \times \exp(\beta_1 X_1) \times \cdots \times \exp(\beta_k X_k).$$

The log link is a natural choice for a positive outcome variable and implies that the covariates affect the mean outcome multiplicatively. Specifically, if X_j is a binary covariate then:

$$\frac{E(Y \mid X_j = 1)}{E(Y \mid X_j = 0)} = \exp(\beta_j),$$

and this interpretation applies for any one-unit change in X_j if it is a continuous covariate. We could, in principle, consider a different link function. For example, if we wanted to model additive effects of the covariates on the mean cost, we could use an identity link. But we would want to make sure that an additive effect was a reasonable choice given the wide range typically spanned by health cost outcomes.

Table 6.3 gives the results of a gamma regression with log link fit to the MEPS 2017 data on total medical expenditures with prior diagnosis of diabetes as the covariate of interest and adjustment for (scaled) age, sex, and race/ethnicity. The result of a linear regression of the log of total medical expenditures adjusted for the same covariates is shown for comparison. Only individuals with positive expenditures are included in these analyses.

As discussed above, the regression coefficients are interpreted as additive effects on the log scale, which translate into multiplicative effects on the original scale. The intercept is the log of the expected costs of the reference group when all (possibly scaled) continuous covariates are zero. In Table 6.3, the reference group is non-Hispanic white men age 18 years who have no prior diagnosis of diabetes, and their average expected cost is exp(7.954) = \$2847. The coefficient of age (0.021) means that each additional year of age over 18 years multiplies the expected costs by exp(0.021) = 1.021, so, for example, a person 40 years old is expected to have $\exp(22 \times 0.021) = 1.021^{22} = 1.587$ times the costs of a similar person aged 18 years. Thus, the expected cost of a non-Hispanic white man aged 40 years who has no prior diagnosis of diabetes is 1.587 × \$2847 = \$4518.

In the gamma model with log link, the multiplicative effects of a covariate are interpreted conditional on the other covariates being fixed but do not depend on their specific values. The coefficient of the indicator of prior diabetes diagnosis is 0.701, implying that the average medical expenditures among participants with a prior diabetes diagnosis are exp(0.701) = 2.016 higher than the average medical expenditures among participants with the same age, sex, and race/ethnicity but without a prior diagnosis. The expected cost of a non-Hispanic white man age

Table 6.3 Fitted linear regression of the log of positive total medical expenditures and gamma regression of total medical expenditures using a log link in MEPS 2017 for participants age 18 years or older adjusted for age, sex, and race/ethnicity

Model	Variable	Coefficient	SE	*P*-value
Gamma	Intercept	7.954	0.052	< 0.001
Gamma	Age−18	0.021	0.001	< 0.001
Gamma	Sex = female	0.203	0.040	< 0.001
Gamma	Race = Hispanic	−0.250	0.051	< 0.001
Gamma	Race = non-Hispanic black	−0.129	0.057	0.02
Gamma	Race = non-Hispanic mixed/other	−0.264	0.071	< 0.001
Gamma	Diabetes = yes	0.701	0.059	< 0.001
Lognormal	Intercept	6.593	0.030	< 0.001
Lognormal	Age−18	0.027	0.001	< 0.001
Lognormal	Sex = female	0.353	0.023	< 0.001
Lognormal	Race = Hispanic	−0.615	0.030	< 0.001
Lognormal	Race = non-Hispanic black	−0.398	0.033	< 0.001
Lognormal	Race = non-Hispanic mixed/other	−0.426	0.042	< 0.001
Lognormal	Diabetes = yes	0.930	0.034	< 0.001

18 years with a prior diagnosis is therefore $2.016 \times \$2847 = \$5750$ and for a non-Hispanic white man aged 40 years with a prior diagnosis is $2.016 \times \$4518 = \$9108$.

Lest there is any confusion about the difference between the gamma regression and the lognormal regression discussed here, note that in gamma regression the log transformation is applied to the mean cost (Y), affecting only how the mean relates to the covariates. Consequently, in the gamma regression, we simply apply the exponential function to the linear predictor to estimate the (multiplicative) effects of covariates on the mean cost. In contrast, in lognormal regression, the log transformation is applied to the Y values themselves (the mean plus the error term), affecting the entire outcome distribution. To recover the effects of covariates on the mean of Y, we apply the exponential function to the linear predictor, but we have to account for the residual variance when this differs across covariate values [11].

Comparison of the two models via standard measures such as the Akaike Information Criterion or Bayesian Information Criterion is not possible because they are not fit to outcomes measured on the same scale. While the lognormal distribution can accommodate a heavier-tailed outcome than the gamma, the two models are often not distinguishable on the basis of observed data, which may not have many events in the extreme tails of the distribution. However, if interest centers on understanding and predicting these extremes, the two models may yield different results.

In sum, because of its ease of use and interpretability, the gamma regression has become an acceptable and even preferred alternative to the lognormal as a regression framework for estimating mean health care costs. In the next section, we harness this model as one of the components of a model for cost outcomes that include zeros.

6.5 Including the Zeros: The Two-Part Model

In the histograms in Fig. 6.1, there are spikes at zero, reflecting the large fractions of participants that did not use the health care system in 2017. The reasons for this feature of the health cost distribution may be manifold; for example, individuals may be healthy enough that they did not need health care, or they may not have had access to care for reasons related to income or insurance. Regardless of the reasons behind it, the resulting shape of a distribution that includes many zeros may warrant special attention. We call this type of distribution a *mixture* distribution because it reflects outcomes from distinct sub-populations, each with its own underlying component distribution.

It is instructive to spend a moment contemplating how mixture distributions work. In general, if the outcome Y follows a mixture distribution, then a certain fraction of observations (p) follows one distribution (let's call this F with mean μ_F), and the other fraction ($1 - p$) follows another distribution (let's call this G with mean μ_G). Figure 6.4 shows mixtures of two normal distributions ($N(0, 1)$ and $N(5, 3)$) with different mixing probabilities p (0.2 and 0.7). In either panel, the mean of the mixture distribution is intermediate between the means of the component distributions.

When we sample values of a mixture random variable Y, we expect that a fraction p will have mean μ_F and a fraction $1 - p$ will have mean μ_G. It follows, then, that the overall mean will be given by:

$$p \times \mu_F + (1 - p) \times \mu_G. \tag{6.4}$$

In Fig. 6.4, the mixing probability $p = 0.2$ leads to a mean of $0.2 \times 0 + 0.8 \times 5 = 4$, and the mixing probability $p = 0.7$ leads to a mean of $0.7 \times 0 + 0.3 \times 5 = 1.5$.

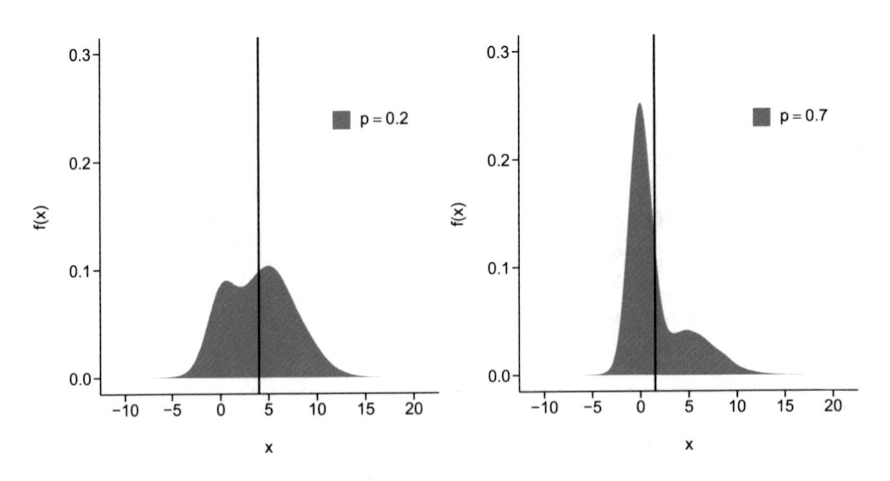

Fig. 6.4 Mixtures of two normal distributions—$N(0, 1)$ and $N(5, 3)$—with mixture probabilities $p = 0.2$ and $p = 0.7$. The black vertical lines show the means of the mixture distributions

In the case of a cost distribution in which a fraction p has non-zero costs and the rest have zero costs, the distribution F consists entirely of positive outcomes, and the distribution G consists entirely of zeros, so the mean μ_G is zero. Consequently, the overall mean is given by $p \times \mu_F$.

When the cost distribution is a mixture of zero and non-zero costs as in Fig. 6.1, standard linear regression methods permit unbiased estimation of the covariate effects on mean costs. However, there is a concern that such methods might lead to inaccurate inferences due to the non-normality of the cost distribution caused by the large number of persons with zero costs—in addition to the skewed distribution of the non-zero costs. Two-part models [13, 14] provide an approach that accommodates both the spike at zero and the right skewness of the non-zero costs while still enabling estimation of marginal covariate effects on mean costs.

The key to understanding two-part models is to recognize the two-component nature of the cost-generating mechanism that leads to mixture distributions such as those shown in Fig. 6.1. The first component reflects whether a person accesses the system and incurs costs, and this part is captured in the two-part model using a binary random variable Z with $Z = 0$ for zero costs and $Z = 1$ for non-zero costs. The second component is the cost-generation process for persons with non-zero costs, and this part is captured in the two-part model using a right-skewed random variable Y. The two-part model estimates the effect of a covariate X on both the probability of having non-zero costs ($p = P(Z = 1)$) and the mean cost among persons with non-zero costs ($\mu = E(Y)$). Then it combines the results to produce an estimate of the effect of X on the overall mean cost, which according to Eq. (6.4) is given by $p \times \mu$.

In the MEPS diabetes analysis, we use logistic regression (see Chap. 4) to model the indicator of non-zero expenditures among all participants and a gamma regression (Sect. 6.4) to model the mean expenditures among participants with non-zero expenditures. This yields a linear model for logit(p) and a linear model for log(μ). Adjusting both models for (scaled) age, sex, and race/ethnicity, the estimated coefficients for each model are presented in Table 6.4, which indicates that not only does a prior diabetes diagnosis increase the mean costs among persons who incurred costs, as shown in the gamma regression, but it also increases the odds of incurring costs by a factor of $\exp(1.85) = 6.30$.

The two-part model [14] enables a rich understanding of the effect of covariates on costs by interrogating both the chance of incurring costs (also referred to as *extensive margins* [8]) and the magnitude of the costs if non-zero (*intensive margins*).

The logistic part models the probability that different groups will have non-zero costs. For example, the probability that a non-Hispanic white man age 40 years without a prior diagnosis of diabetes has non-zero costs is:

$$\frac{\exp(0.732 + 22 \times 0.033)}{1 + \exp(0.732 + 22 \times 0.033)} = 0.811,$$

Table 6.4 Fitted two-part model for total medical expenditures in MEPS 2017 for participants age 18 years or older adjusted for age, sex, and race/ethnicity

Model	Predictor	Coefficient	SE	*P*-value
Logistic	Intercept	0.732	0.045	< 0.001
Logistic	Age−18	0.033	0.001	< 0.001
Logistic	Sex = female	0.843	0.037	< 0.001
Logistic	Race = Hispanic	−1.202	0.044	< 0.001
Logistic	Race = non-Hispanic black	−0.856	0.053	< 0.001
Logistic	Race = non-Hispanic mixed/other	−0.716	0.064	< 0.001
Logistic	Diabetes = yes	1.854	0.122	< 0.001
Gamma	Intercept	7.954	0.052	< 0.001
Gamma	Age−18	0.021	0.001	< 0.001
Gamma	Sex = female	0.203	0.040	< 0.001
Gamma	Race = Hispanic	−0.250	0.051	< 0.001
Gamma	Race = non-Hispanic black	−0.129	0.057	0.02
Gamma	Race = non-Hispanic mixed/other	−0.264	0.071	< 0.001
Gamma	Diabetes = yes	0.701	0.059	< 0.001

while the corresponding probability for a counterpart with a prior diagnosis is:

$$\frac{\exp(0.732 + 22 \times 0.033 + 1.854)}{1 + \exp(0.732 + 22 \times 0.033 + 1.854)} = 0.965.$$

How do we put the two parts in Table 6.4 together? The key is to recognize that the overall mean cost is $p \times \mu$. Using the calculations above, the average cost for a non-Hispanic white man age 40 years with no prior diagnosis of diabetes is $0.811 \times \$4518 = \$3664$, while the average cost for a counterpart with a prior diagnosis is $0.965 \times \$9108 = \$8789$. Thus, for a non-Hispanic white man age 40 years, prior diagnosis of diabetes is associated with an average increase in costs of $\$8789 - \$3664 = \$5125$ or $\$8789/\$3664 = 2.4$-fold higher costs.

Now we've seen how to interpret the estimated coefficients in each part of a two-part model and how to calculate average costs for specific individuals in a way that accounts for the component with zero costs, but how can we summarize the overall effect of a covariate on mean costs? To calculate this, we leverage the technique of *recycled predictions* for estimation of marginal effects, which we presented in Chap. 4 as a method for estimating *marginal additive effects* from non-linear models like logistic regression.

To recap, the marginal additive effect associated with a binary covariate like prior diagnosis of diabetes is calculated from the fitted regression model as follows. First, we use the model to predict the outcome after setting the diabetes indicator to 0 for all subjects. Then, we use the model to predict the outcome after setting the diabetes indicator to 1 for all subjects. Finally, we average the within-subject differences between the two predicted outcomes.

In Chap. 4, we explained that the marginal (adjusted) additive effect of a covariate X on an outcome Y was interpretable as the expected absolute change in $E(Y)$ associated with a one-unit change in X adjusted for the other covariates and averaged over their joint distribution in the data. We can similarly define a marginal (adjusted) multiplicative effect, which would be interpreted as the expected *relative* change in cost associated with a prior diabetes diagnosis, again adjusted for the other covariates and averaged over their joint distribution in the data.

In the two-part model, the mixture formulation tells us that the overall mean of Y is $p \times \mu$. If we want to predict the effect of a prior diabetes diagnosis on $p \times \mu$, we can leverage recycled predictions to do it. We use the fitted models to predict $p \times \mu$, setting the diabetes covariate first to 0 and then to 1 for every person. To estimate the marginal adjusted additive effect, we average the within-subject differences between the two predictions; to estimate the marginal adjusted multiplicative effect, we average the within-subject ratios. Formally, we can enumerate the steps in the procedure as follows:

1. Set the binary covariate X to 0 for all individuals, and use the fitted models to predict $\widehat{p}_0 = P(Y = 1 \mid X = 0)$ and $\widehat{\mu}_0 = E(Y \mid X = 0)$ keeping the other covariates as observed.
2. Set the binary covariate X to 1 for all individuals, and use the fitted models to predict $\widehat{p}_1 = P(Y = 1 \mid X = 1)$ and $\widehat{\mu}_1 = E(Y \mid X = 1)$ keeping the other covariates as observed.
3. For the marginal adjusted additive effect, compute:

$$\text{average}(\widehat{p}_1 \times \widehat{\mu}_1 - \widehat{p}_0 \times \widehat{\mu}_0).$$

For the marginal adjusted multiplicative effect, compute:

$$\text{average}\left(\frac{\widehat{p}_1 \times \widehat{\mu}_1}{\widehat{p}_0 \times \widehat{\mu}_0}\right).$$

In this procedure, the $\widehat{p}$ values are predictions from the logistic regression fit to the indicator of non-zero expenditures, and the $\widehat{\mu}$ values are predictions from the gamma regression fit to the fraction of the sample with non-zero expenditures. Even though this latter model is fit only to a subset of the sample, it is used to predict expenditures for the whole sample. This makes an implicit assumption, namely, that if individuals with zero costs could incur costs, they would do so similarly to those individuals who actually had non-zero costs. Subject to this caveat, the procedure provides a coherent estimate of the marginal effect of a diabetes diagnosis on the mean cost after adjusting for the other covariates and accounting for the spike at zero in the observed cost distribution.

When we use recycled predictions to estimate marginal effects of diabetes on the mean annual health care costs in the MEPS 2017 data, we find the marginal additive effect is \$6560 and the marginal multiplicative effect is 2.48. The standard errors of these estimates depend on the standard errors of the marginal probability and marginal mean estimates from the two component models; we explain how to use bootstrapping to obtain standard errors for marginal effect estimates from two-part models in Chap. 7.

Our results indicate that a prior diabetes diagnosis is estimated to inflate a subject's annual medical expenditures by $6560 and by a factor of 2.48. As a check on the marginal additive effect, we often use the result from a standard linear regression model of cost adjusting for the same covariates; in this case, the result is $7059. The linear regression fit obviously does not account for the non-normal features of the observed expenditures, but it provides an unbiased estimate of the marginal adjusted additive effect of a diabetes diagnosis on mean costs and is helpful as a rough confirmation of the validity of the recycled prediction result. Unfortunately, there is no similar simple model to check the marginal multiplicative effect for a two-part model.

It is reasonable to ask what the value of a two-part model might be if we are ultimately going to fold the two parts together into a result about the marginal mean cost. There are several reasons why understanding the approach and being able to implement it are important. First, this approach accommodates the awkward distributional features of mixture cost distributions that have a spike at zero. Ignoring these features and using a standard linear regression model could lead to inferences that are not correct and that either underestimate or overestimate the uncertainty in the parameter estimates. Second, and perhaps even more useful, the two-part model provides insight into the mechanism underlying any observed differences in the marginal mean cost. Specifically, it allows us to understand whether differences in the marginal mean are associated with the differences in the likelihood of incurring costs, in the costs themselves, or both. In the example studied in this chapter, we found that a prior diabetes diagnosis increased the odds of non-zero medical expenditures and also increased the magnitude of the expenditures. Thus, diabetes was a significant factor in both parts of the model, and both parts contributed to its effect on the marginal overall mean cost.

6.6 Beyond Mean Costs

Up to this point, this chapter has focused on regression methods for modeling the mean of health cost outcomes. However, for skewed data, the mean is not always the best descriptive measure, and certain scientific questions might be better addressed by summarizing the outcome in terms of the median. The median is not sensitive to extreme values (either zero costs or large costs), and it gives a more representative summary of the typical costs of a group. And—in contrast with mean costs—the log of the median cost is also the median of the log cost.

Consider again the linear regression we fit to the log of total medical expenditures among MEPS 2017 adult participants with positive expenditures in Table 6.3. The coefficient for a prior diabetes diagnosis (0.93) reflects the estimated multiplicative effect of a prior diabetes diagnosis on the mean of log expenditures. We encountered challenges when we back-transformed this estimate by exponentiating it due to having to account for heteroskedasticity. But these challenges are avoided if we interpret the result as the estimated effect on median costs. If $\log(Y)$ is

Table 6.5 Median regression for total medical expenditures in MEPS 2017 for participants age 18 years or older. Results are reported separately for all participants and for participants with non-zero medical expenditures

Group	Variable	Coefficient	SE	*P*-value
Overall	Intercept	374.89	41.97	< 0.001
Overall	Age−18	41.17	1.20	< 0.001
Overall	Sex = female	518.20	27.94	< 0.001
Overall	Race = Hispanic	−934.26	40.33	< 0.001
Overall	Race = non-Hispanic black	−678.94	46.09	< 0.001
Overall	Race = non-Hispanic mixed/other	−751.66	45.60	< 0.001
Overall	Diabetes = yes	4215.40	203.14	< 0.001
Non-zero costs	Intercept	617.21	52.81	< 0.001
Non-zero costs	Age−18	48.85	1.55	< 0.001
Non-zero costs	Sex = female	569.26	43.97	< 0.001
Non-zero costs	Race = Hispanic	−952.32	52.36	< 0.001
Non-zero costs	Race = non-Hispanic black	−684.63	74.88	< 0.001
Non-zero costs	Race = non-Hispanic mixed/other	−789.69	65.28	< 0.001
Non-zero costs	Diabetes = yes	3852.05	208.13	< 0.001

approximately normally distributed (actually we only need the distribution of Y to be symmetric), then the mean of $\log(Y)$ is also the median of $\log(Y)$ and is equal to the log of the median of Y. Further, the log is an increasing function and therefore preserves the ordering of values, so when we exponentiate the log of median of Y, we get back the median of Y. In other words, if log-transformed costs really are approximately normally distributed, then we can draw valid inference using a log cost model but interpreting the exponentiated results in terms of median costs.

Using this interpretation, we estimate that median expenditures among participants with positive expenditures and a prior diabetes diagnosis are $\exp(0.93) = 2.53$ times the median expenditures among participants without a prior diagnosis. From Table 6.3, we can calculate a 95% confidence interval for this multiplicative effect as $\exp(0.93 \pm 1.96 \times 0.034) = (2.37, 2.71)$.

Alternatively, as discussed in Chap. 3, we can fit a model directly to the median to obtain an additive effect estimate without relying on the log transformation or the normal assumption. This amounts to fitting:

$$\text{median}(Y) = \beta_0 + \beta_1 X_1 + \cdots + \beta_k X_k,$$

and interpreting the β coefficients as the difference in median dollars for a one-unit change in the corresponding covariate.

Table 6.5 presents the results of median regressions fitted only to participants with positive costs and also to the whole sample, including participants with zero costs. A prior diabetes diagnosis is associated with a $4215 higher median cost overall and a $3852 higher median cost when restricted to individuals with positive costs. The effect of a prior diabetes diagnosis on the median is smaller than the effect on the mean because the median is less sensitive to participants with high medical costs. In general, the quantile regression approach is agnostic to the spike at zero and permits "thinking beyond the mean" [15] when appropriate.

In conclusion, the analyst studying health expenditures can select from a range of modeling options for both the non-zero component of the expenditure distribution and the probability that expenditures are positive. When there is a spike at zero, a two-part model may provide more insight into reasons for any observed marginal effects than a model that does not acknowledge the mixture nature of the outcome. For modeling positive expenditures, a lognormal model was historically the approach of choice, but a GLM like the gamma model is now frequently preferred. Manning and Mullahy [16] provide a detailed discussion of the considerations involved when choosing between the two and offer a guide for when it may be preferable to use a lognormal rather than a gamma GLM model despite the retransformation issue [11].

A version of the two-part model that applies to count outcomes is called the hurdle model. Deb and Norton [8] use both a two-part model for expenditures and hurdle models for office-based and emergency department visits to comprehensively describe the changes in young adult expenditure patterns following the Affordable Care Act young adult expansion. Ultimately, the final model should be informed by the objective of the analysis and selected to maximize the chance that it will produce a valid and interpretable result.

6.7 Software and Data

R code to download data and to carry out the examples in this book is available at the GitHub page https://roman-gulati.github.io/statistics-for-health-data-science/. In addition to the R packages cited in Chap. 1, this chapter also used the `lmtest` [17] and `quantreg` [18] packages. A package for two-part modeling, `twopm` [14], is available in Stata and estimates marginal additive effects along with standard errors.

References

1. Arora, V., Moriates, C., Shah, N.: The challenge of understanding health care costs and charges. AMA J. Ethics **17**, 1046–1052 (2015)
2. Brownlee, S., Colucci, J., Walsh, T.: What health care costs really means. The Atlantic (2012). https://www.theatlantic.com/health/archive/2012/12/what-health-care-costs-really-means/266522/

3. Agency for Healthcare Research and Quality: Medical Expenditure Panel Survey (). http://www.ahrq.gov/research/data/meps/index.html. Accessed 12 Feb 2020
4. Gaskin, D.J., Richard, P.: The economic costs of pain in the United States. J. Pain **13**, 715–724 (2012)
5. Biemer, A., Cawley, J., Meyerhofer, C.: The high and rising costs of obesity to the US health care system. J. Gen. Internal Med. **32**, 6–8 (2017)
6. Kim, D., Basu, A.: Estimating the medical care costs of obesity in the United States: systematic review, meta-analysis, and empirical analysis. Value Health **19**, 602–613 (2018)
7. Kirkland, E.B., Heincelman, N., Bishu, K.G., Schumann, S.O., Schreiner, A., Axon, R.N., Mauldin, P.D., Moran, W.P.: Trends in healthcare expenditures among US adults with hypertension: National estimates, 2003–2014. J. Am. Heart Assoc. e008731 (2018)
8. Deb, P., Norton, E.C.: Modeling health care expenditures and use. Annu. Rev. Public Health **39**, 489–505 (2018)
9. For Disease Control, C., Prevention: National Diabetes Statistics Report, 2020 (2020)
10. Association, A.D.: Economic costs of diabetes in the U.S. in 2017. Diabetes Care **41**, 917–928 (2018)
11. Manning, W.G.: The logged dependent variable, heteroscedasticity, and the retransformation problem. J. Health Econ. **17**, 283–295 (1998)
12. Breusch, T.S., Pagan, A.R.: A simple test for heteroscedasticity and random coefficient variation. Econometrica **47**, 1287–1294 (1979)
13. Deb, P., Norton, E.C., Manning, W.G.: Health Econometrics Using Stata. Stata Press, College Station (2017)
14. Belotti, F., Deb, P., Manning, W.G., Norton, E.C.: twopm: two-part models. STATA J. **15**(1), 3–20 (2015)
15. Lê Cook, B., Manning, W.G.: Thinking beyond the mean: a practical guide for using quantile regression methods for health services research. Shanghai Arch. Psychiatry **25**(1), 55 (2013)
16. Manning, W.G., Mullahy, J.: Estimating log models: to transform or not to transform? J. Health Econ. **20**, 461–494 (2001)
17. Zeileis, A., Hothorn, T.: Diagnostic checking in regression relationships. R News **2**(3), 7–10 (2002). https://CRAN.R-project.org/doc/Rnews/
18. Koenker, R.: quantreg: Quantile regression (2019). https://CRAN.R-project.org/package=quantreg. R package version 5.52

Chapter 7
Bootstrap Methods

Abstract Sample data provide information about a population, but this information is subject to uncertainty due to the sampling process. Statistical uncertainty is most often quantified in terms of standard errors or confidence intervals, which are traditionally estimated based on formal mathematical derivations. With increasing growth in and access to computational power, computationally based algorithms have been developed to quantify uncertainty and to test hypotheses. Instead of relying on theoretical understanding of the uncertainty of the sampling process and the properties of statistical estimators, these algorithms "bootstrap" or repeatedly resample from the observed data to quantify uncertainty. In a wide range of settings, this approach has been shown to be reliable, and it may be even more intuitive than classical methods. This chapter explains the bootstrap technique and applies it to calculate the variance of the estimates of marginal effects in a two-part model of health care costs.

7.1 Uncertainty and Inference in Statistical Models

Statistics has been called the science of uncertainty; it provides a quantitative framework for understanding how reliably we can learn about a process of interest from (noisy) data. In practice, statistical results are based on samples, and estimates are ideally reported together with measures of their uncertainty. These measures include standard errors, confidence intervals, and p-values. The traditional way of understanding uncertainty in an estimate is in terms of the variability of the estimate if the sampling could be repeated many times. This is referred to as a *frequentist* statistical perspective.

We begin this chapter with a short review of measures of uncertainty because this provides a natural starting point to introduce a modern alternative approach to obtaining them, namely, bootstrapping.

Consider the objective of estimating average yearly medical expenditures among adults living in the United States. To learn about this quantity, we might take a random sample of 10,000 persons, or we might stratify by state and take a random sample of 200 persons from each. Either way, we will record the year's medical

R. Etzioni et al., *Statistics for Health Data Science*, Springer Texts in Statistics,
https://doi.org/10.1007/978-3-030-59889-1_7

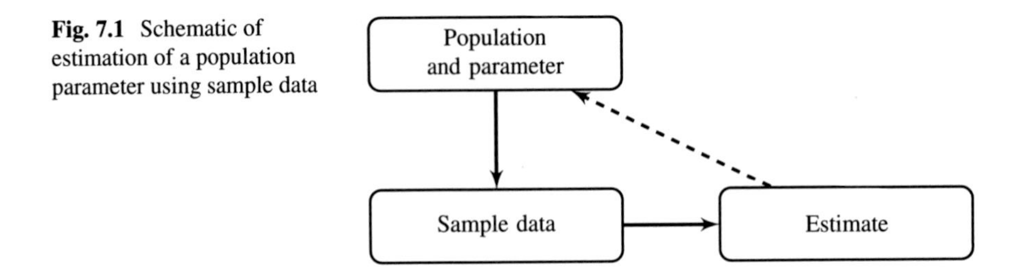

Fig. 7.1 Schematic of estimation of a population parameter using sample data

expenditures for each sampled person and, based on this information, estimate the mean expenditure using a simple average over the sample or, if we stratified by state, using a weighted average taking the state population sizes into account. The general procedure is visualized in the flowchart in Fig. 7.1.

In words, we start by defining the population and parameter of interest, then we collect sample data according to a specified sampling design, and finally we estimate the quantity of interest using the data collected. In general, the sample estimate will not exactly match the corresponding population parameter; rather, there will be a discrepancy between the two quantities because the estimate was calculated using the sample instead of using the whole population. If another sample was drawn from the same population, the new estimate would not be the same as the previous one. This variation in the estimate is a manifestation of its uncertainty. Whenever we approximate a population parameter based on an estimate from a sample, and we want to make an inference about the population based on the estimate, we must acknowledge this uncertainty.

A traditional measure of uncertainty is the standard error. This is a classical mathematical measure that summarizes the variability of an estimate, but its meaning is not totally transparent. An alternative is a confidence interval, which translates the variability in an estimate into an uncertainty interval around it. If the statistical problem involves hypothesis testing, we might calculate a p-value, which uses the variability (again) of the estimate to determine whether it is atypical under a specified null hypothesis.

So what is the variability of an estimate and how does it capture uncertainty?

According to frequentist reasoning, the uncertainty of a statistical estimate can be measured by considering a large (theoretically infinite) number of repetitions of the sampling and estimation procedures. Thus, if instead of a single sample we took many samples using exactly the same sampling design (say, a random sample of 200 persons from each state) and calculated the estimate in exactly the same way (a weighted average based on state population sizes), then we would end up with a collection of estimates that were each obtained from the same procedure. The uncertainty of the estimate would be reflected by how widely its values fluctuated from sample to sample. The variability is a specific measure of the uncertainty given by the average squared deviation of the sample estimates from their mean. The standard error is the square root of this measure of variability, and it is equivalent to the standard deviation of the estimates in the collection.

How might we use this reasoning to obtain the standard error of the average yearly medical expenditures based on a sample of 200 persons from each state? If we follow the steps above, then, instead of taking a single sample, we would take a large number N of samples, each containing 200 persons from each state, obtain N estimates of the average cost, and report the standard deviation of these estimates as the standard error of our estimate. While this would provide a valid result, the effort and resources needed would be prohibitive.

Can we mimic this approach and calculate the standard error using a single sample? It turns out that for this and many similar problems, computational approaches have been developed for precisely this purpose. These approaches tend to be computationally intensive, replacing repeated sampling of individuals in the real-world population with repeated sampling of individuals in a virtual population created using the sample data. The approaches occupy a critical niche, particularly in complex estimation settings where standard errors of estimates cannot easily be calculated mathematically or where mathematical formulas produce poor approximations. Such settings include estimation of marginal covariate effects in two-part regression models for health care costs (Chap. 6) and population surveys, which typically use complex sampling including stratification and clustering (Chap. 9). The advances represented by these computationally intensive methods are hard to overstate, as they have permitted valid inferences to be drawn in these and countless other settings.

In this chapter, we will focus on one of these computational approaches—the bootstrap method—and illustrate how to use it for statistical inference: variance estimation, confidence interval construction, and statistical testing. For a more complete and formal introduction to the bootstrap, see Efron and Tibshirani [1, 2].

7.2 The Bootstrap for Variance Estimation

Bootstrapping was first suggested by Bradley Efron in his seminal paper *Bootstrap Methods: Another Look at the Jackknife* [3]. Efron's logic was extremely simple: If a sample is a trustworthy representation of a population, then let's pretend that it is the population. In other words, replace repeated sampling from the real-world population with repeated sampling from our sample. In principle, we are replacing the population data distribution with the sample distribution.

We demonstrate the bootstrap approach using sample data on yearly medical expenditures. For pedagogical purposes, we use Medical Expenditure Panel Survey (MEPS) data among persons age 18 years or older in the year 2017 as the total population and select at random 2000 records to represent our sample. MEPS is an annual rolling panel survey of the civilian non-institutionalized US population [4]. It collects information on socio-demographics, health conditions, insurance coverage, and medical costs. At the end of this chapter, we comment on the implications of applying bootstrap methods to data sampled using complex sampling designs, such as MEPS and other national surveys.

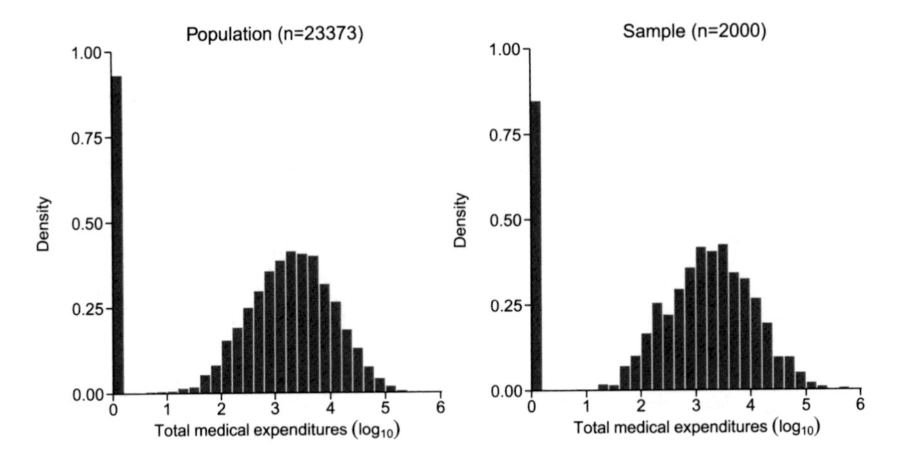

Fig. 7.2 Histograms of total medical expenditures ($\log_{10}$ scale) among persons age 18 years or older in MEPS 2017 data ("Population") and in the random sample ("Sample")

Figure 7.2 shows histograms of total medical expenditures for adults in the MEPS 2017 sample ("Population") on the left and in a random sample of 2000 records on the right ("Sample"). Because the original distribution is skewed to the right, the histograms are represented using a log (base 10) scale, and \$1 was added to all costs before transforming to avoid taking the log of zero. The distribution in the sample closely resembles the distribution in the population with modest differences: the sample distribution is less smooth, and a smaller fraction is represented by the lowest bin. The skewed distribution of the data and the large number of zeros suggest that the median may be a more appropriate summary measure than the mean. The sample median cost is $\widehat{M} = \$1180$ (median $\log_{10}(\text{cost} + \$1) = 3.07$). How can we obtain a standard error for this estimate to quantify its uncertainty?

The bootstrap procedure uses the histogram of the Sample on the right side of Fig. 7.2 as the true distribution of costs in the population, repeatedly draws new samples from the observations that generated this histogram, and uses the medians of the new samples drawn to quantify the uncertainty in $\widehat{M}$.

Formally, the steps in the bootstrap algorithm are as follows:

1. Draw a large number (B) of "bootstrap" samples from the original sample. Each bootstrap sample has the same number of observations as in the original sample, and it is drawn by randomly sampling with replacement.
2. For each sample, calculate the statistic of interest (in our example, the median $\widehat{M}$). This yields a collection of B bootstrap estimates of the statistic.
3. Use the B bootstrap estimates of the statistic to calculate a measure of the statistic's uncertainty (e.g., a standard error).

Why do we draw bootstrap samples with replacement? Because we are using the sample data distribution as an approximation to the population data distribution. As we draw observations from the sample, we replace them so as not to change the

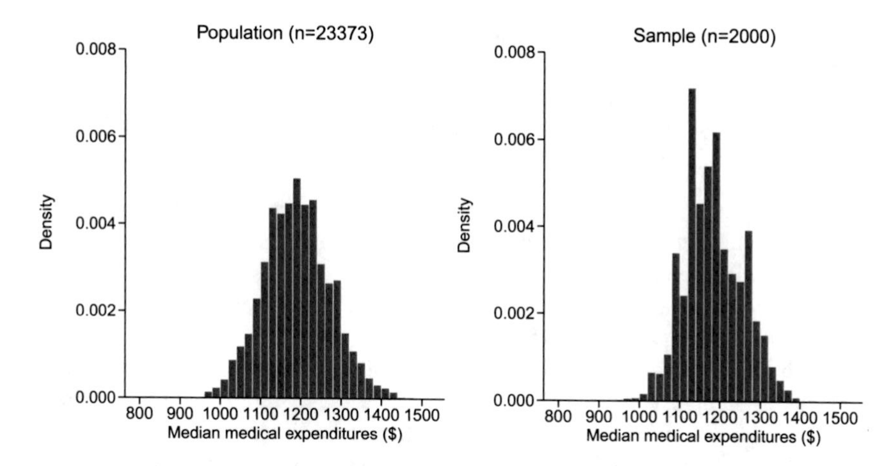

Fig. 7.3 Histograms of median medical expenditures ($) obtained in 5000 bootstrap samples from the original sample ($n = 2000$) from MEPS 2017 data ("Population") and from the random sample ("Sample")

distribution. If we did not sample with replacement, we would end up with each bootstrap sample being identical to the original sample.

A histogram of the medians of $B = 5000$ bootstrap samples is shown on the right in Fig. 7.3, where cost is now presented on the original scale of US dollars. Although the original sample is quite large, comprising 2000 observations, the median estimate is still prone to statistical uncertainty reflected by the variability of the medians of the bootstrap samples. The distribution is symmetric and has a bell-like shape centered around the estimated median of $1189, but the estimates vary from $970 to $1566. The standard error is given by the standard deviation of the bootstrapped medians, which is found to be $76.

It is worth appreciating how natural it is to estimate the standard error in this way and how faithful it is to the frequentist reasoning described in Sect. 7.1. The frequentist approach defines the uncertainty of an estimate in terms of its fluctuation across repeated samples from the same population. This is exactly what bootstrapping does: it repeatedly samples from the same "population," and the collection of estimates obtained from each sample is then used to directly quantify uncertainty. The only caveat is that the "population" here is the original sample and not the underlying population.

Given that we are drawing from the sample, which is much smaller than the population, how do we know that we are adequately capturing the uncertainty in $\widehat{M}$? In the current example, we use a graphic to suggest that this is likely to be the case when the original sample is relatively large. The left side of Fig. 7.3 shows the distribution of the median costs based on 5000 samples of 2000 persons each from the MEPS 2017 data. The right side of Fig. 7.3 shows that the histogram obtained by resampling datasets from the original sample with $n = 2000$ is quite similar. However, if the original sample was small (e.g., $n = 50$), this would not be guaranteed.

Based on the preceding discussion, we can observe that the following conditions are needed for the bootstrap algorithm to reliably measure the uncertainty around a statistic:

1. The sample should accurately represent the population. Fortunately, for a large enough sample (several hundred observations is generally sufficient), this condition is often satisfied.
2. There should be a large number of resamplings. Fortunately, this is not an issue with current computing capabilities.
3. The bootstrap should recapitulate the sampling process. In other words, the bootstrap samples must be drawn in the same way the original sample was drawn, following the same sampling design. If the original sample was drawn using stratification, the bootstrap sample should do the same. Similarly, the estimation procedure should be the same.

In our example, the first condition appears to be satisfied because the histograms in Fig. 7.2 are similar. The second and third conditions are also satisfied because the bootstrap samples were randomly drawn and the calculation of the median was consistently applied.

The bootstrap approach to quantify uncertainty is not limited to simple statistics like the median; it can be used in more complex settings. For example, suppose we want to estimate the proportion of persons in a group who will have no medical expenditures in a certain year. We know the age and sex of each person, and suppose the probability of a person having no medical expenditures is well approximated using logistic regression (Chap. 4). For concreteness, let $i = 1, \ldots, m$ index subjects, and let Y_i denote the event of no medical costs during the year, so $Y_i = 1$ if there are no costs and $Y_i = 0$ if there are costs. Our statistic of interest is the proportion of persons with no costs: $\bar{Y} = (1/m) \sum_{i=1}^{m} Y_i$. Because the probability of having no costs depends on subject-specific covariates (viz., age and sex), the proportion $\bar{Y}$ is a complicated statistic with expectation given by:

$$\bar{\pi} = \frac{1}{m} \sum_{i=1}^{m} \frac{\exp(\beta_0 + \beta_1 \text{age}_i + \beta_2 \text{sex}_i)}{1 + \exp(\beta_0 + \beta_1 \text{age}_i + \beta_2 \text{sex}_i)}, \tag{7.1}$$

where age_i and sex_i are the age (in years) and an indicator of sex (0 for men and 1 for women) for subject i and β_0, β_1, and β_2 are the coefficients in the logistic model.

To estimate $\bar{\pi}$, we can first fit a logistic regression to the original sample and then use the estimated coefficients to calculate Eq. (7.1). The uncertainty around the resulting estimate depends on the uncertainty in the estimated coefficients, and calculating it mathematically requires non-trivial derivations and programming. Bootstrap variance estimation is a simple and attractive alternative.

Table 7.1 shows the fitted logistic regression. The negative coefficients for age and sex indicate that the odds of no costs decreases with age and is smaller for

Table 7.1 Fitted logistic regression of no medical expenditures based on a sample of 2000 persons age 18 years or older in the MEPS 2017 data with maximum likelihood and bootstrap standard errors (SEs) based on 5000 bootstrap samples

Predictor	Coefficient	Maximum likelihood SE	Bootstrap SE
Intercept	0.6370	0.1778	0.1630
Age	−0.0433	0.0040	0.0034
Sex = female	−0.7782	0.1271	0.1300

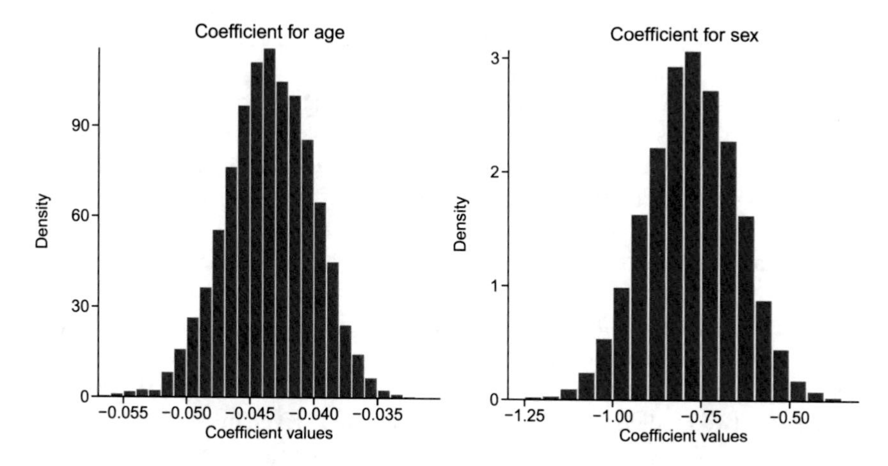

Fig. 7.4 Histograms of coefficients for age and sex from logistic regressions for no medical costs fit to 5000 bootstrap samples from an original sample of 2000 persons age 18 years or older drawn from the MEPS 2017 data

women than for men. The maximum likelihood standard error (SE) is shown for each coefficient, and bootstrap estimates based on $B = 5000$ bootstrap samples are also shown. To produce the bootstrap estimates, we fit the logistic regression to each bootstrap sample, stored the estimated coefficients, and calculated standard deviations over the 5000 sets of stored coefficients. The two different estimates of the standard errors are very similar. Figure 7.4 shows histograms of the bootstrap estimates of the coefficients for age and sex and shows that they are approximately normally distributed, supporting maximum likelihood theory that the coefficient estimates are normally distributed in sufficiently large samples. In such scenarios, we expect the bootstrap and maximum likelihood estimates of standard errors to be close.

While the bootstrap is not really needed for coefficient standard errors, since maximum-likelihood-based standard errors are generally produced with regression output, this is not always the case. For derived quantities like the proportion $\bar{\pi}$ in Eq. (7.1), and for marginal effects of covariates (see Sect. 4.6.2), maximum likelihood estimates of standard errors are not automatically calculated (though routines have recently become available for the latter). We show how to use the bootstrap to produce standard errors for marginal effects.

As discussed in Chap. 5 (for the case of logistic regression, see Sect. 4.6), marginal effects are useful in generalized linear models when the link function g is not the identity function. In these models, the linear predictor applies not to the mean of the outcome but to a non-linear function of the mean. In logistic regression, for example, the linear predictor linear regression applies to the logit of the mean ($g(\pi) = \text{logit}(\pi) = \log[\pi/(1-\pi)]$). A consequence of this formulation is that adjusted coefficient estimates are interpretable in terms of changes in $g(\pi)$ rather than changes in the probability π.

In the present example, if the coefficient of sex in the logistic regression is β_2, then this implies that the logit(π) for women is β_2 greater than the logit(π) for men. If we want to know how π differs for women, then, because the logit function is non-linear, the answer depends on the other covariates in the model (in this case, age). Indeed, the expected change in π for women versus men may differ for older versus younger subjects. We say that the estimated effect of sex on π is conditional on age.

Marginal effects average conditional effects over the distribution of the other covariates in the sample to produce estimates of covariate effects on the probability scale π rather than on logit(π). The marginal additive effect of sex on π is estimated by setting sex to 1 and predicting π for all subjects ($\widehat{\pi}_{1i}$) and then setting sex to 0 and predicting π once again ($\widehat{\pi}_{0i}$). The marginal additive effect averages the difference between the two predictions for each individual and is given by:

$$\text{MAE} = \frac{1}{m}\sum_{i=1}^{m}(\widehat{\pi}_{1i} - \widehat{\pi}_{0i}).$$

The MAE for sex in our sample is -0.10; in words, we estimate that women have a 10% lower probability of having no medical costs compared to men. To quantify uncertainty around this estimate, we can calculate a standard error using the 5000 bootstrap samples that generated the estimated coefficients shown in Fig. 7.4. Within each bootstrap sample, we use the corresponding coefficient estimates to produce a value for MAE. A histogram of the bootstrap values of MAE is shown in Fig. 7.5; the standard deviation of these bootstrap values, and our standard error for the MAE, is 0.02.

The computing time needed to calculate the bootstrap estimate was less than 1 min on a modern laptop. There was no need to derive new mathematical results, and only basic programming was required; we say "basic" because it is straightforward to take advantage of built-in functions to repeatedly draw samples and fit regressions.

The bootstrap can be used to derive the standard error of almost any statistic of interest, and this flexibility is testament to the power of the bootstrap approach. Let's see how we might apply it to the two-part model for annual health care costs studied in Chap. 6. In that example, we used the MEPS 2017 data to estimate the effect of a diabetes diagnosis on mean medical expenditures for the year. For simplicity, we restricted to adult subjects with non-missing diabetes status. We used

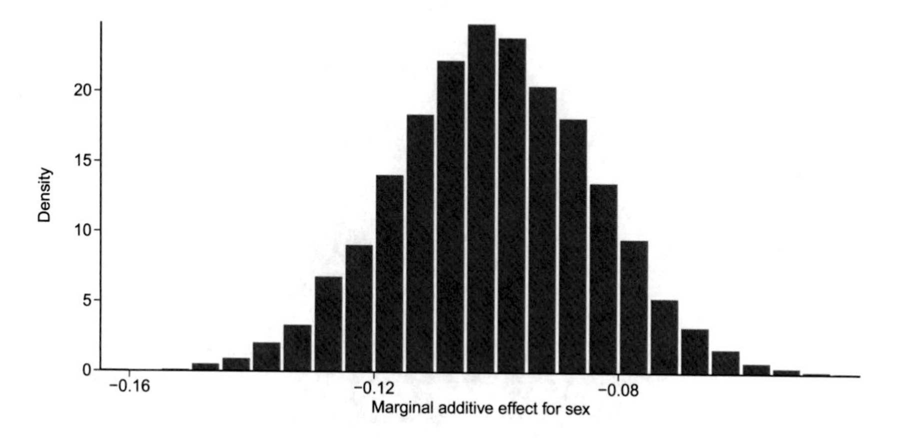

Fig. 7.5 Histogram of marginal additive effects for sex on the probability of no medical expenditures from 5000 bootstrap samples from the original sample ($n = 2000$) from MEPS 2017 data

logistic regression to model the probability of non-zero expenditures (p) and a gamma regression to model the mean expenditures (μ) for persons with positive expenditures, adjusting both models for (scaled) age, sex, and race/ethnicity.

In this two-part model, the overall mean cost was $p \times \mu$. For the marginal (adjusted) additive effect of diabetes on the overall mean health care cost, we computed:

$$\text{average}(\hat{p}_1 \times \hat{\mu}_1) - \text{average}(\hat{p}_0 \times \hat{\mu}_0), \tag{7.2}$$

where a subscript 1 indicates predictions from each submodel after setting the diabetes covariate to 1 and a subscript 0 indicates predictions after setting the diabetes covariate to 0. Based on this expression, we estimated that diabetes increased the expected annual health care cost by $6560.

To bootstrap the standard error, we now draw 1000 bootstrap samples from the MEPS 2017 data. Within each sample, we fit the two regression models that constitute the two-part model and calculate the marginal additive effect according to Eq. (7.2).

Figure 7.6 shows a histogram of the results. The standard deviation of the marginal additive effect across the bootstrap samples is $546, and this is our bootstrap standard error.

7.3 Bootstrap Confidence Intervals

Bootstrapping permits several different ways of constructing confidence intervals. When the bootstrapped statistics are normal, bootstrap standard errors can be

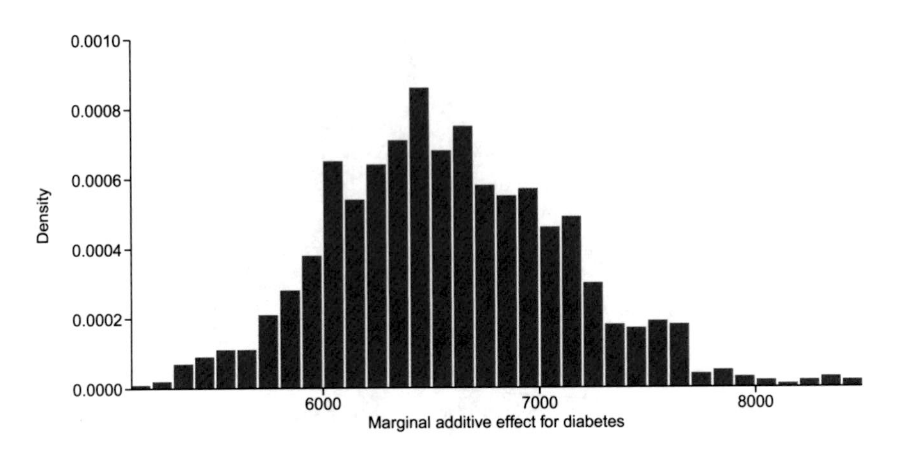

Fig. 7.6 Histogram of marginal additive effects for diabetes on annual medical expenditures from 1000 bootstrap samples of MEPS 2017 data for participants age 18 years or older adjusted for age, sex, and race/ethnicity

Table 7.2 Bootstrap-t and bootstrap percentile 95% confidence intervals for logistic regression coefficients and median medical expenditures based on a sample of 2000 persons age 18 years or older in the MEPS 2017 data

Parameter	Estimate	Bootstrap SE	Bootstrap-t	Bootstrap percentile
Intercept	0.637	0.163	(0.317, 0.957)	(0.333, 0.964)
Age	−0.043	0.003	(−0.050, −0.037)	(−0.050, −0.037)
Sex = female	−0.778	0.130	(−1.033, −0.523)	(−1.038, −0.529)
Median cost	1180	73	(1037, 1323)	(1059, 1327)
Probability of no costs	0.169	0.008	(0.153, 0.186)	(0.154, 0.187)

used to construct normal-based confidence intervals, sometimes called bootstrap-t confidence intervals. For a confidence level of $(1 - \alpha) \times 100\%$, a normal bootstrap confidence interval takes the form:

$$\text{Estimate} \pm z_{1-\alpha/2} \times \text{Bootstrap SE}. \tag{7.3}$$

Here, "Estimate" is the estimate of the quantity of interest from the original sample, and $z_{1-\alpha/2}$ is the upper quantile of the standard normal distribution corresponding to a tail probability of $\alpha/2$.

Figures 7.3, 7.4, and 7.5 indicate that it might be reasonable to use a normal bootstrap confidence interval for the sample median and the marginal additive effect of sex on the probability of having no medical expenditures. Table 7.2 shows 95% bootstrap confidence intervals calculated using formula (7.3).

A second type of bootstrap confidence interval, the bootstrap percentile interval, does not make any assumptions about normality. Instead, it uses the B bootstrap estimates and calculates the $(1 - \alpha) \times 100\%$ central values. This requires sorting the bootstrap estimates from smallest to largest and then using the $\alpha/2 \times B$ and

$(1 - \alpha/2) \times B$ replicates for the lower and upper confidence limits. For example, with $\alpha = 0.05$ and $B = 5000$, these would be the 125th and 4875th observations. This approach does not require the bootstrap distribution to be approximately normal; instead, it directly estimates the limits of the confidence interval using the empirical distribution of bootstrap results. If the distribution of the bootstrap results is approximately normal, then the bootstrap percentile interval is close to the normal-based bootstrap interval. This is indeed the case for the logistic regression coefficients and the marginal additive effect of sex on the probability of no costs (Table 7.2). The distribution of bootstrap estimates of the median cost (right panel in Fig. 7.3) is slightly skewed to the right, causing the small difference between the two intervals.

While both the normal-based and the percentile intervals are intuitive and simple to apply, they may not perform well, and their actual coverage probability may not be as advertised in some settings. For instance, the percentile-based confidence interval may be overly narrow, especially in small samples. Therefore, there are a number of alternative bootstrap confidence interval formulations. Carpenter and Bithell [5] provide a comprehensive review of different options with their properties. For large sample sizes and common estimators, the normal-based and the percentile intervals usually perform well and are generally considered to be valid.

7.4 Hypothesis Testing

The bootstrap can be used to test statistical hypotheses as well. Simple hypotheses can be tested by checking whether a hypothesized value is included in a bootstrap confidence interval. For example, to test whether having no medical expenditures differs by sex in the MEPS 2017 data, we can check whether the bootstrap confidence interval for the coefficient of sex in Table 7.2 includes zero. Because the bootstrap 95% confidence interval (−1.03, −0.52) excludes 0, we reject the null hypothesis at the 5% significance level. In fact, we could also use the bootstrap standard error to generate a test statistic by calculating the standardized variable $Z = \text{Estimate}/\text{Bootstrap SE} = -0.778/0.130 = -5.98$ and referencing it against a standard normal distribution; this gives a p-value < 0.0001.

Bootstrap methods can be applied to test more general hypotheses, such as tests for the independence of two variables. For example, suppose we want to test the hypothesis that annual health expenditures for persons with a prior diagnosis of diabetes and a prior diagnosis of arthritis do not depend on the specific diagnosis. In our sample, there are 383 and 130 persons with a diagnosis of diabetes and arthritis, respectively, after excluding persons with both conditions.

Table 7.3 summarizes the data on expenditures within the two groups as a contingency table. The first two rows show observed numbers of persons (Obs) with expenditures falling within specified intervals that span the range of expenditures. The last two rows show the expected numbers of persons (Exp) in each interval under the null hypothesis: expenditure distributions do not differ in the two group,

Table 7.3 Observed and expected counts of persons with prior diagnosis of diabetes or arthritis based on a sample of 2000 persons from the MEPS 2017 data

Statistic	Group	< \$500	\$500–\$9999	\$1000–\$4999	\$5000–\$99999	≥ \$10000
Observed	Diabetes	23	9	38	21	39
Observed	Arthritis	52	27	142	68	94
Expected	Diabetes	19.01	9.12	45.61	22.55	33.70
Expected	Arthritis	55.99	26.88	134.39	66.45	99.30

or, equivalently, condition and expenditures are independent. The expected numbers are the product of the marginal probabilities times the sample size; for example, the expected number of persons with diabetes and medical costs < \$500 is the marginal probability of having a prior diabetes diagnosis (130/(383+130)) times the marginal probability of having medical costs < \$500 (75/(383+130)) times the sample size (383+130).

A popular test statistic for contingency tables sums the squared standardized differences, $Q = \sum(\text{Exp} - \text{Obs})^2/\text{Exp}$. Calculating this statistic for our data, we obtain $Q = 4.1$. Does this indicate different distributions, or is this statistic compatible with the null hypothesis? We can answer this question by calculating a p-value using the bootstrap. The p-value would be the probability of obtaining a test statistic Q greater than or equal to the observed value 4.1 *when the data follow the null model.*

To calculate a p-value using a bootstrap, we need to resample in a manner that reflects the null hypothesis. This is a little different than our previous use of the bootstrap to quantify variability. In that case, we resampled directly from the observed data, replicating the process that generated the original sample. In this case, we must resample from the observed data but in a way that reflects an assumption of independence between expenditures and diagnosis. This assumption is equivalent to assuming that the distribution of expenditures is the same in the two groups. But if this were the case, then we would be able to consider all of the observations in both groups as being from a single large group. Recognizing this is the key to a procedure for bootstrapping in this case. The steps are as follows:

1. Pool the 383 and 130 observations from the diabetes and arthritis groups. Then, sample 383 (representing diabetes) and 130 (representing arthritis) observations with replacement from the pooled data. This provides bootstrap samples with the same numbers of observations in the two groups as in the original data, but now forced to have the same distribution.
2. Repeat this sampling procedure B times; each time, calculate the statistic Q.
3. Calculate the p-value as the proportion of Q values greater than or equal to 4.1.

The left side of Fig. 7.7 shows a histogram of Q values obtained by applying the bootstrap algorithm with $B = 5000$ replications. The vertical line shows the observed value of the test statistic $Q = 4.1$, and the bootstrap p-value is the area in the tail of the histogram to the right of this value. The p-value is 0.40, so there is no evidence that the distributions of expenditures (at least as summarized in the table)

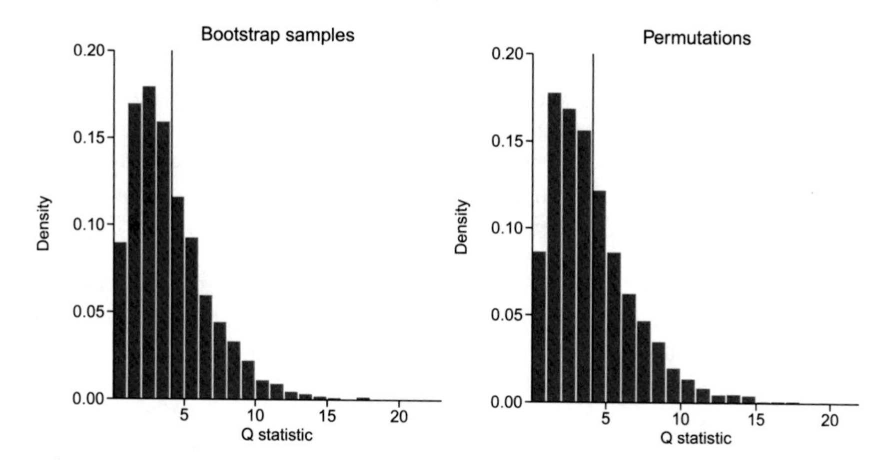

Fig. 7.7 Histograms of the Q statistic from 5000 bootstrap samples and from 5000 permutations. The vertical lines show the observed Q statistic; the p-value is the area to the right of this line

differ in these two groups. In fact, Q is a well-studied statistic used for frequency tables, which under the null hypothesis has approximately a χ^2 distribution with (in this example with 5 expenditure strata) 4 degrees of freedom. The theoretical p-value is 0.39, which almost exactly recapitulates the p-value from the bootstrap.

In this example, by construction, the bootstrap algorithm guarantees that samples are drawn so that the two groups (diabetes and arthritis patients) have the same distribution. However, the bootstrap distribution is only an approximation to the data distribution, and it is not useful in the case of small samples. An alternative is a method called permutation testing, which is also valid for small sample sizes.

A permutation test evaluates the comparability of outcomes across subgroups in a sample. A permutation is simply a random shuffling of the group labels so that the outcome (here, expenditures) for each subject remains the same, but the group label may be changed (from diabetes to arthritis or vice versa). If the null hypothesis holds and the medical condition is independent of expenditures, this shuffling should not affect the distribution of the test statistic Q. If we know the values of expenditures in our sample and we know the number of individuals in each of the groups, any permutation of the group labels is equally likely under the null hypothesis. Therefore, the permutation test replaces the first step in the bootstrap algorithm with:

1′. Randomly permute (shuffle) the group labels. This yields a permutation sample with the same number of observations in the two groups as in the original data.

The other two steps remain exactly the same as in the bootstrap p-value computation. Note that, in contrast to a bootstrap sample, the values of expenditures in the replicate samples do not change.

The right side of Fig. 7.7 shows the test statistic obtained from $B = 5000$ permutations of the data. The p-value is given by the area of the histogram to the right of 4.1 and is calculated to be 0.40. The bootstrap and permutation tests produce similar null histograms for Q and result in similar p-values.

Permutation tests can be applied to compare any summary of interest across groups. If, for example, interest focuses on comparing the mean, rather than the distribution of the outcome, the permutation test would follow the same reshuffling procedure but each time the difference (Δ) in group means would be calculated. At the end, the observed difference in group means would be compared against a histogram of the Δs across the permutations.

Because permutation tests are easy to perform and are valid for small samples, they are more broadly applicable than bootstrap-based tests so long as the research question can be formulated as a comparison of groups. In most other settings, particularly those with large samples, bootstrap-based tests are likely to be preferred.

7.5 Summary

The bootstrap approach is a powerful method for statistical inference, permitting assessment of uncertainty when standard estimation procedures are not applicable or when estimates are complex. Despite its intuitive nature, however, the bootstrap has some caveats. First, it is only as representative of the population as the original sample. If the original sample is selective, the bootstrap will produce a similarly selective result. Further, if the original sample is small, then the bootstrap will be limited in its ability to represent the tails of the data distribution and could underestimate the variability of the statistic of interest.

The bootstrap procedure presented in this chapter makes no assumptions about the data-generating mechanism. Formally, this is called the non-parametric bootstrap; a parametric bootstrap generates data from a specified distribution. The non-parametric bootstrap preserves not only the distribution of the outcome in the original sample but also the distribution of the covariates and their associations with one another and with the outcome.

It is important to remember that resampling (and hence bootstrapping) is a stochastic endeavor. If two people run the same bootstrap routine, they will generally not obtain identical results. The variation across bootstrap results is called Monte Carlo variation, and it is more pronounced when the number of replications is small. The recommended number of bootstrap replications has evolved (and grown) over time from 1000 to 2000 replications to more than 10,000. The number of replications needed to achieve stable results in the presence of Monte Carlo variation will depend on the specific data structure and data properties in any given application. Hesterberg [6] recommends that at least 10,000 replications be performed.

The bootstrapping procedure must preserve the original design of the study that yielded the sample. If the data are clustered, then a bootstrapping procedure that preserves the cluster structure must be used (i.e., the procedure should sample clusters rather than individuals). Bootstrapping data collected under complex designs, such as survey data, requires special treatment because the data do not represent the population and random sampling from the observations does not imitate the sampling mechanism.

Since the bootstrap was first introduced, hundreds of papers have been published that seek to refine and improve on the basic idea. Only the basic idea is illustrated in this chapter; refinements and modifications that address possible biases in the estimates or confidence intervals are not considered. To read more about these refinements, including alternative bootstrap confidence intervals that address possible biases, see Efron and Tibshirani [2] and Efron and Hastie [7].

In conclusion, the bootstrap represents a significant advance for the analyst utilizing complex methods or conducting inference when the assumptions underlying standard procedures are questionable. A general principle is that bootstrap resampling needs to preserve the study design and replicate the full variability of the sampled data. There is a right way—and plenty of wrong ways—to bootstrap in any setting.

7.6 Software and Data

R code to download data and to carry out the examples in this book is available at the GitHub page https://roman-gulati.github.io/statistics-for-health-data-science/. In addition to the R packages cited in Chap. 1, this chapter also used the `rsample` package [8].

References

1. Efron, B., Tibshirani, R.J.: Bootstrap methods for standard errors, confidence intervals, and other measures of statistical accuracy. Statist. Sci. **1**, 54–75 (1986)
2. Efron, B., Tibshirani, R.J.: An Introduction to the Bootstrap. CRC Press, Boca Raton (1994)
3. Efron, B.: Bootstrap methods: another look at the jackknife. Ann. Statist. **7**(1), 1–26 (1979)
4. Agency for Healthcare Research and Quality: Medical expenditure panel survey (2020). http://www.ahrq.gov/research/data/meps/index.html. Accessed Feb. 12 2020
5. Carpenter, J., Bithell, J.: Bootstrap confidence intervals: when, which, what? A practical guide for medical statisticians. Statist. Med. **19**, 1141–1164 (2000)
6. Hesterberg, T.C.: What teachers should know about the bootstrap: resampling in the undergraduate statistics curriculum. Am. Statist. **69**(4), 371–386 (2015)
7. Efron, B., Hastie, T.: Computer Age Statistical Inference: Algorithms, Evidence and Data Science. Cambridge University Press/IMS Monographs, Cambridge (2016)
8. Kuhn, M., Chow, F., Wickham, H.: rsample: general resampling infrastructure (2020). https://CRAN.R-project.org/package=rsample. R package version 0.0.6

Chapter 8
Causal Inference

Abstract This chapter introduces the concept of causality, going beyond association to learn how change in a treatment or an exposure leads to a change in the outcome. Causal effects are ideally investigated via randomized controlled trials, but such studies cannot address all health care questions of interest. Consequently, observational data sources are increasingly being used to answer causal questions. This chapter reviews the challenges of using observational studies for causal inference and presents several approaches designed to address these challenges. The chapter is divided into three parts. First, we introduce the potential problems and biases that can arise when using observational data for causal questions. We then describe causal graphs as a vehicle for representing biological or clinical knowledge in a way that reveals the causal structure and informs analysis. Finally, we work through the steps involved in translating from causal graphs to regression analyses and describe several methods, including propensity score approaches, for making causal inferences from observational data.

8.1 Introduction

Can a new medicine improve the prognosis of a disease? Does preventing smoking reduce the risk of a lung cancer diagnosis and, if so, by how much? How will lower-premium high-deductible health insurance plans impact health expenditures? These questions go beyond simple association to the effects of interventions and policy changes on health outcomes. They are what-if questions ("What if we change exposures or processes?"). They are causal questions, focusing on the extent to which a specific exposure or intervention is responsible for a specific consequence, and answering them requires causal inference.

Consider the question of smoking and lung cancer. Many studies have shown that people who smoke have a higher risk of developing lung cancer. By itself, this is evidence of an association between smoking and lung cancer. To make the leap from this observation to being able to recommend stopping smoking in order to lower lung cancer risk requires showing that the association is causal.

R. Etzioni et al., *Statistics for Health Data Science*, Springer Texts in Statistics,
https://doi.org/10.1007/978-3-030-59889-1_8

The study of causality focuses on how changing an input X, such as stopping smoking, affects an output Y, such as a lung cancer diagnosis; the answer has direct implications regarding potential interventions to reduce disease burden and improve population health.

The most widely accepted and commonly used method to establish causal effects is the randomized trial. Most comparative (Phase III) randomized trials involve hundreds or thousands of patients across multiple centers. Large sample sizes help ensure that any observed effect is real and not a result of chance alone. Randomization of participants to treatment groups helps ensure that the groups are generally comparable in all aspects except the treatment.

Randomized trials are expensive and often lengthy. Further, they are only appropriate for addressing questions that do not pose significant logistical and ethical issues. In particular, the principle of equipoise dictates that a patient may be ethically enrolled into a randomized trial only if adequate uncertainty exists regarding which of the treatments being compared is likely to be superior. Consequently, randomized trials can only be used to estimate causal effects in a limited range of settings.

Observational studies that utilize large national surveys or registries can also be used to estimate causal effects. Indeed, much of comparative effectiveness research aims to support evidence-based decisions using observational data. However, using observational data to learn about causal effects is tricky because randomization is replaced by selection; subjects are assigned to different treatments or interventions by self-selection or by their physician, based on their medical status.

Confounding by indication refers to bias due to imbalance of variables between comparison groups that affect both the cause and the outcome. In such settings, observed effects may be driven by the confounders and not by the cause. This was exactly the reasoning of Sir Ronald A. Fisher, one of the most influential statisticians of the twentieth century, who supported tobacco companies in their fight against the accusation that smoking caused lung cancer. Fisher's argument was that the association might be a result of a genetic confounder that predisposed individuals to smoke and also made them susceptible to lung cancer [1]: "any statistical association, observed without the precautions of a definite experiment, always allow ... that cigarette-smoking and lung cancer, though not mutually causative, are both influenced by a common cause, in this case the individual genotype."

Fisher was correct in his claim—a confounder can theoretically explain any observed association between two variables. Yet it is now widely accepted that smoking causes lung cancer; this acceptance comes partly from experimental evidence of biological effects but also partly from rigorous study of observational data.

This chapter addresses methods for making causal inferences from observational data. We present a general framework that uses graphs to translate causal questions into regression equations in realistic observational settings. Work in this area has expanded rapidly in the last several decades with contributions from statistics, epidemiology, computer science, economics, and the social sciences.

At the level of the individual, the causal effect is the answer to a counterfactual question. For example, for a lung cancer patient with a long history of smoking, what would have happened if, contrary to fact, he had never smoked? Would he have been diagnosed with lung cancer? Different individuals may be affected differently by exposures like tobacco smoke, so we will focus on estimating the average causal effect in a population. We cover stratifying, matching, and weighting as methods to address confounding and selection bias, and we introduce propensity scores as a tool to estimate the average causal effect in complex problems with multiple confounders. The theory that connects the average causal effect with the formal philosophical framework of counterfactuals or potential outcomes is briefly summarized at the end of the chapter.

8.2 Simpson's Paradox

In randomized trials with no missing data, the average causal effect is simply estimated as the difference in the average outcomes in the intervention and control groups. However, in observational studies, such a simple approach can be biased or even misleading. A surprisingly common scenario is the bias highlighted by *Simpson's paradox*. This paradox is foundational to understanding one of the key challenges to conducting causal inference using observational data.

To illustrate Simpson's paradox, we use an analysis of the cost-effectiveness of three treatments for kidney stones [2]. In this observational study, patients were assigned to treatments by physicians without randomization. Here we focus on two of the treatments—open surgery ($n = 350$) and percutaneous nephrolithotomy (PCNL, $n = 350$)—with overall success rates of 78.0% and 82.6%, respectively, as shown in the rightmost column of Table 8.1. This simple comparison seems to indicate better outcomes for kidney stones treated with PCNL.

However, when patients are stratified according to the size of their stones, as shown in the middle two columns of Table 8.1, we find better outcomes for both small and large kidney stones treated with open surgery. In contrast with the marginal analysis, the stratified analysis supports open surgery for all patients.

This phenomenon, where an advantage is observed for one treatment when examining overall outcomes but a disadvantage for that treatment is observed when conditioning on another variable, is known as Simpson's paradox. (*Conditioning* on a variable means conducting separate analyses for different levels of that variable.) In this example, stone size is a *confounder*—a variable that affects both the treatment selected and the likelihood of success—and it is the reason for the paradox.

Table 8.1 Success of treatments for kidney stones

Treatment	Small (<2 cm)	Large (≥2 cm)	Total
Open surgery	81/87 (93.1%)	192/263 (73.0%)	273/350 (78.0%)
PCNL	234/270 (86.7%)	55/80 (68.8%)	289/350 (82.6%)
Total	315/357 (88.2%)	247/343 (72.0%)	562/700 (80.3%)

Simpson's paradox occurred here because the proportions of patients with large stones were not the same in the two groups. About 75% of open surgery patients and 23% of PCNL patients had large stones. Large stones are harder to treat and are associated with a lower success rate. Consequently, overall, open surgery seems inferior, but within groups defined by stone size, a clearer picture of its efficacy relative to PCNL emerges. While such an unbalanced distribution of a confounder is unlikely in randomized trials, it is common in observational studies and cannot be ignored if causal inference is the objective of the analysis. In observational studies, we always have to ask: "What else could be going on?"

8.3 Causal Graphs

Real-world observational data analyses are invariably complex. Even if the question at hand is relatively straightforward (e.g., "Is one treatment superior to another?" or "Does exposure to a certain chemical make people more likely to develop a certain disease?"), other variables affecting the outcome or the selection mechanism must be explicitly considered when formulating the analytic model.

Simpson's paradox demonstrates the importance of considering confounders when conducting causal inference. In this section, we examine the general problem of considering causal relationships between variables in a conceptual model and translating the conceptual model into an analytic model. In later sections we will use the analytic model to estimate causal effects.

Causal graphs are key to systematically accounting for relevant variables in the analysis. In particular, *directed acyclic graphs* (DAGs) can be used to represent a conceptual model of variables and their causal relationships. In principle, DAGs can be constructed without any knowledge of statistics or probability, and statisticians can analyze DAGs without any subject-matter background. Thus, DAGs form a critical meeting place for researchers from different disciplines to interact around a scientific question. Statistical methods, guided by causal graphs, can estimate causal effects reliably only if the graph is a faithful reflection of reality. For this reason, the first and probably the most important step in causal inference is building a causal graph.

A DAG connects two related variables with an arrow indicating the direction of causality. Thus an arrow from X to Y indicates that X has a direct effect on Y, so that a change in X causes a change in Y. It is implicit in this setting that X must occur before Y, so the arrow also indicates the direction of time.

The simplest interesting DAGs contain three variables and two arrows. We examine these foundational DAGs in the following subsections. In all the DAGs considered, the scientific question is about the causal effect of X on Y, but there is another variable, denoted Z, that is related to both X and Y.

8.3.1 Confounders

Figure 8.1 presents the DAG for Z as a confounder.

Confounding occurs when there is a variable that causes both X and Y. In this scenario, Z induces an association between X and Y even if X does not cause Y. In other words, even though there is no arrow between X and Y, there will be an association between them due to their common dependence on Z.

We saw confounding in the example of treatments for kidney stones in Sect. 8.2. In that example, X is treatment (open surgery or PCNL), Y is outcome (success or not), and Z is stone size (small or large), which affected both the choice of treatment and the chance of success. In that example, however, there was also evidence of an arrow directly connecting X to Y.

Whether or not X causes Y, the true effect of X on Y will not be correctly estimated if we do not account for the effect of any and all confounders Z in the analysis. Indeed, in the kidney stone example, PCNL is the preferred treatment when stone size is ignored, but open surgery is preferred when stone size is taken into account. Conversely, if there were no real advantage for open surgery, we should see similar success rates when stone size is taken into account. Basically, conditioning on stone size restricts comparisons of the two treatments to patients with similar stone sizes, thereby isolating the effect of treatment choice on the outcome. In a sense, we remove the effect of stone size from the analysis by accounting for it via conditioning.

Confounding is unavoidable and must be addressed whenever observational data are analyzed. It is the primary reason why we cannot, in general, make causal inferences from observational data and why we always have to question whether there may be other explanations for an association between a covariate and an outcome. The good news is that, in principle, if we are able to identify and observe all confounders, we should be able to remove their effects from the analysis and validly draw causal inferences. The bad news is that, in practice, there might always be unknown confounders. Consequently, when building a DAG, one should be thoroughly familiar with the research setting and identify all confounders affecting

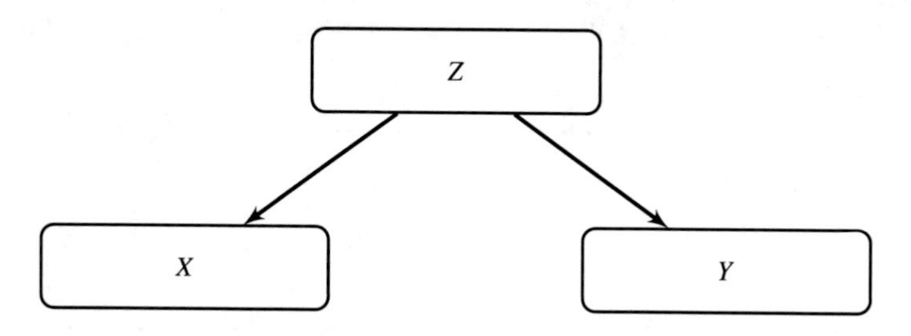

Fig. 8.1 The confounder Z causes both X and Y

both the cause and effect variables. And this is why, in the kidney stone example, causal conclusions based on the analysis that conditions on stone size are only valid if stone size is the only confounder.

8.3.2 Mediators

Figure 8.2 presents the DAG for Z as a mediator.

Mediation occurs when X affects Y via an intermediate variable Z. For example, a chronic disease (X) may affect the annual days hospitalized (Z), which in turn affects total health expenditures (Y). While the causal effect of X on Y is of primary interest, the identification of a mediator offers an opportunity to understand the mechanism driving the effect. The analysis will be determined by the scientific objective—understanding the causal effect of X on Y or understanding the mechanism driving the effect.

In Fig. 8.2, for simplicity, there is no arrow directly connecting X to Y. If there were such an arrow, it would signify that X has a direct (non-mediated) effect in addition to an indirect (mediated) effect on Y. In this case, the analysis will still be determined by the scientific question, but now with the potential distinction between the direct and indirect effects of X on Y.

An example with both direct and indirect effects is the relation between a chronic disease like multiple sclerosis (X) and annual health expenditures (Y). If Z denotes the number of days hospitalized, then X is a cause of Z because individuals with multiple sclerosis tend to be hospitalized more than those without the disease. Further, Z affects Y, as more hospitalization days means more medical costs. An arrow should also be drawn directly from X to Y in this example, as multiple sclerosis patients are prescribed medications that directly affect their medical expenditures. Here one may be more interested in the total effect of multiple sclerosis on medical expenditures, and the direct effect that excludes costs due to hospitalization may be less important.

An interesting example of mediation, discussed in Pearl and Mackenzie [3], is the study of gender discrimination in admissions to the graduate program at the University of California Berkeley in 1973 [4]. This is another example of Simpson's

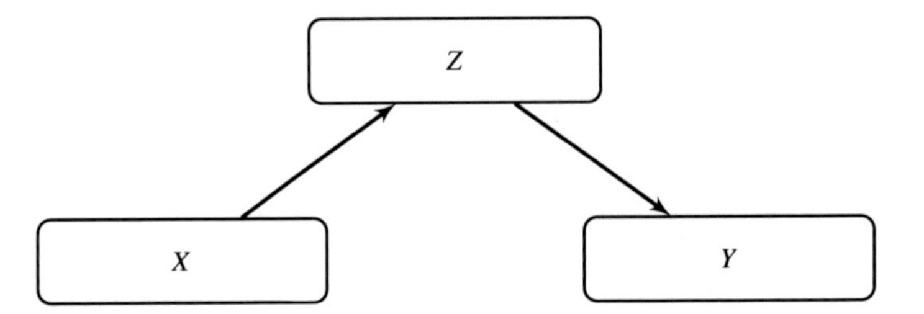

Fig. 8.2 The mediator Z mediates the causal effect of X on Y

paradox, but due to a mediator and not a confounder. Here the variable X is gender and the variable Y is admission to the graduate program. While about 44% of the male applicants were admitted, only 33% of the female applicants were admitted. The question of interest was about the mechanism behind this observed difference: Was it due to gender discrimination (a direct arrow from X to Y)? In fact, there is strong evidence that it was due to a mediator. Recognizing that admission is determined by department, Bickel et al. [4] considered the department as a mediator Z because men and women have different department preferences (the arrow from X to Z) and different departments have different admission rates (the arrow from Z to Y). The question of systemic discrimination is then transformed into a question about the existence of a direct effect from X to Y given the mediator Z. In fact, their findings suggested that such an effect, if it existed, actually favored women.

8.3.3 *Colliders*

Figure 8.3 presents the DAG for Z as a collider.

When both X and Y are causes of a variable Z, we call Z a *collider*. A study of genetic predisposition to nicotine dependence provides an example [5]. Here X is the genotype and Y is a measure of nicotine dependence. Since both genotype and nicotine dependence affect lung cancer (Z), the DAG has arrows from X to Z and from Y to Z, and we call lung cancer a collider for the causal effect of genotype and nicotine dependence.

Note that the DAG in Fig. 8.3 does not contain an arrow from X to Y, meaning in this example there is no causal effect of genotype on nicotine dependence. In fact, since the only relationship between X and Y is via the collider Z, we do not expect any association between X and Y. However, an association will still be found within sub-populations defined by Z. Specifically, if there is a genotype–lung cancer association in addition to a smoking–lung cancer association, we will observe an association between nicotine dependence and genotype within the subgroup of lung cancer patients. This is known as *collider bias*. In effect, by conditioning on the collider, we induce an association between X and Y.

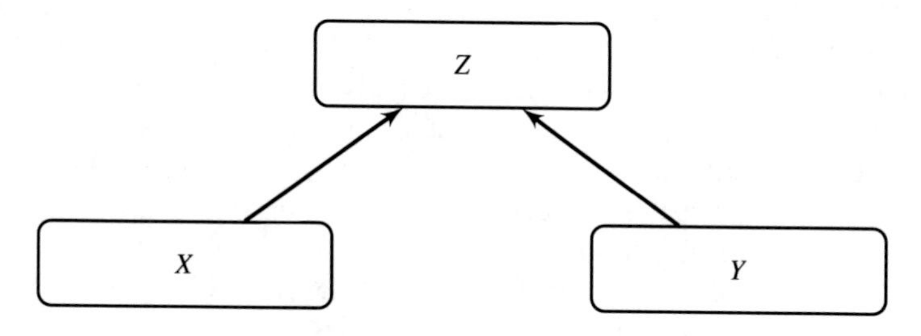

Fig. 8.3 The collider Z is caused by both X and Y

Another example relates collider bias to selection bias. Consider two diseases, such as diabetes and gallbladder inflammation, and the question of whether the former is a cause of the latter. Here, hospitalization plays the role of collider. In terms of Fig. 8.3, X is an indicator of diabetes, Y is an indicator of gallbladder inflammation, and Z is an indicator of hospitalization. Naturally, both diabetes and gallbladder inflammation are causes for hospitalization; hence we will tend to see more individuals having both conditions among hospitalized patients than in the whole population. This will generate a type of selection bias if data are restricted to a sub-population, for example, when study participants are selected from hospital registries or discharge databases. This kind of bias was first identified by Berkson [6] and is named *Berkson's bias*.

While sampling is not a biological or clinical process, and it is therefore somewhat unnatural to include it in the DAG, it can be a good practice to do so. Including sampling in the DAG (as an indicator of sample inclusion for each person in the population), with arrows from all factors determining selection to the sampling indicator, enables accounting not only for confounders but also for selection bias induced by colliders. It might be appropriate for this kind of information to be incorporated by a statistician after a subject-area specialist has developed a pure causal graph.

8.4 Building a Causal Graph

A causal graph is constructed by including the cause X, the outcome Y, and all variables affecting X, Y, or both X and Y, together with arrows connecting all pairs of causally related variables. Ideally, the causal graph should be constructed while planning the study in order to understand which variables are critical to the analysis and should be collected and which can be safely ignored.

As an example, consider the effect of arthritis on health expenditures as shown in Fig. 8.4. The cause (arthritis) and the effect (health expenditures) are in blue to emphasize that the relationship between these variables is the central question of interest. The arrows from the cause to the effect are also in blue, which together summarize the total effect. The pain variable is a mediator, as arthritis causes pain, which increases medical care utilization and costs. Several variables that are associated with arthritis, such as age, sex, and chronic conditions like diabetes, also increase health expenditures. Age is clearly related to arthritis, particularly osteoarthritis, which is much more prevalent in older than in younger patients. Sex is also linked with arthritis since women are more likely to be diagnosed with arthritis than men [7]. And diabetes has been associated with an increased risk of both rheumatoid arthritis and osteoarthritis [8]. The arrows for these variables indicate direction of dependence; for example, a patient's level of pain depends on his/her sex and not the other way around.

In practice, the process of constructing a DAG requires deep subject-area knowledge. The statistician's role is to provide general guidance about implications

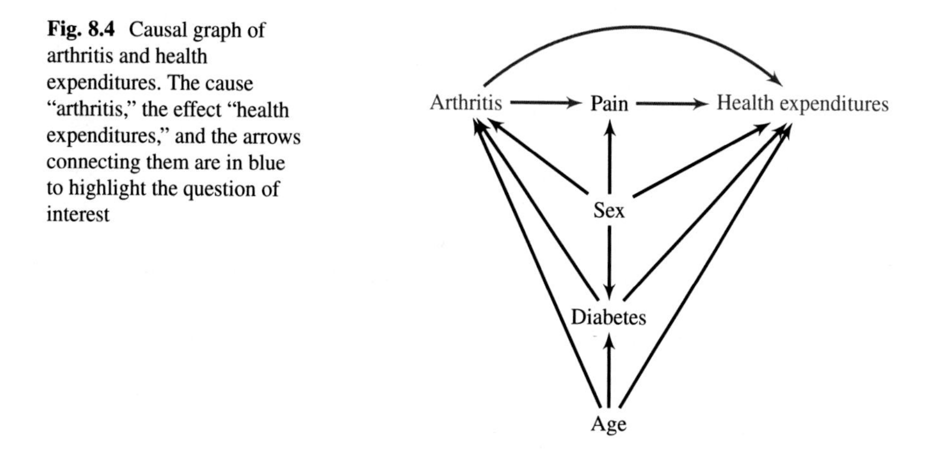

Fig. 8.4 Causal graph of arthritis and health expenditures. The cause "arthritis," the effect "health expenditures," and the arrows connecting them are in blue to highlight the question of interest

of missing variables or incorrectly specified relationships. Note also that the DAG is built for a specific question, for example, the causal effect of arthritis on health expenditures. A different graph would be appropriate if the scientific question concerned the effect of diabetes on health expenditures, say, because related variables may be different from the ones included in Fig. 8.4.

8.5 Estimating the Causal Effect

We are now ready to discuss the statistics of causal inference based on observational data using the causal graph. Informally, we define the *average causal effect* of X on Y as the change in Y induced by a change in X, all other things being equal. We formalize this notion below, but for now our goal is to capture the idea of the change in Y that is driven solely by a change in X and not by other confounders that may themselves be associated with X or Y.

A *path* in a DAG is a set of variables connected by arrows. A *causal path* from X to Y is expressed by a set of arrows starting at X and ending at Y, all pointing in the same direction toward Y. Because of this single-directional flow of influence like water through a pipe, causal paths are referred to as *open paths*. In the arthritis example, the two paths:

$$\text{arthritis} \rightarrow \text{health expenditures}$$

$$\text{arthritis} \rightarrow \text{pain} \rightarrow \text{health expenditures}$$

are the only causal paths (in terms of the scientific question of interest). As in the simple DAGs in Sect. 8.3, a variable that sits in the causal path between X and Y is a mediator that controls the mechanism by which X affects Y. In this example, pain is a mediator that captures some or all of the effect of arthritis on health expenditures.

This example also includes several paths that are not causal (in terms of the scientific question of interest). For example, the paths:

$$\text{arthritis} \leftarrow \text{diabetes} \rightarrow \text{health expenditures} \tag{8.1}$$

$$\text{arthritis} \leftarrow \text{age} \rightarrow \text{diabetes} \leftarrow \text{sex} \rightarrow \text{health expenditures} \tag{8.2}$$

are non-causal paths (in this sense). What distinguishes these paths from a causal path is that their arrows do not all point in the same direction. Indeed, we see two distinct types of non-causal paths.

In paths like (8.1), a variable Z points (directly or indirectly) to X and to Y. This forked structure indicates that Z is a confounder. Like the causal path, it is open in the sense that it induces an association between X and Y. Figure 8.4 contains several non-causal paths having a forked structure, with age, diabetes, and sex each playing the role of Z and confounding the association between arthritis and health expenditures.

In paths like (8.2), a variable Z sits on the path between X and Y, but two arrows point to Z. This inverted fork structure indicates that Z is a collider. In path (8.2), two arrows point to diabetes, showing that it is a collider of the association between arthritis and expenditures. We say that this type of non-causal path is *closed* or *blocked*—there is no indicated association between X and Y through this path.

To estimate the causal effect of X on Y, we need to block all non-causal paths, but without blocking causal paths (we discuss below how to practically block paths—at this point it is important to understand which paths should be blocked). Paths that include colliders are already blocked, but paths that include confounders need to be blocked. Our goal is to achieve a state described as *dependence-separation* or *D-separation*, where all non-causal paths are blocked.

In practice, D-separation can be achieved by conditioning on confounders but not on mediators or colliders. In Fig. 8.4, diabetes is a confounder of the causal relationship between arthritis (X) and health expenditures (Y). By conditioning on diabetes, which covaries with X, we remove its effect from the X–Y relationship, thereby isolating the effect of arthritis on expenditures. In the same figure, pain is a mediator of the X–Y relationship. We don't want to adjust for pain because this would remove part of the effect of arthritis on health expenditures. Finally, diabetes is a collider, and conditioning on it in the analysis can induce a spurious association between X and Y. In DAG jargon, we say that adjusting for a collider Z *opens a path* between X and Y because it induces an association between these variables. Thus, if we must include a collider in the analysis (e.g., because it is also a confounder, which is the case with diabetes in this example), our only recourse is to block the path another way.

Going back to Fig. 8.4 then, we recommended controlling for diabetes as it is a confounder on a non-causal path (8.1); however, this opens non-causal path (8.2) that was originally blocked due to diabetes being a collider. To re-block non-causal path (8.2), we should also control for age or sex (or both) since these variables are also on this path. In fact, in this example, controlling for age, sex, and diabetes blocks all non-causal paths and enables us to estimate the causal effect of arthritis on health expenditures under the model represented by Fig. 8.4. Lederer et al. [9] make the general point that in a complex DAG, such as the one in Fig. 8.4, a small number of variables (a "minimum set" of confounders) will often block most substantial non-causal paths.

Blocking all non-causal paths in the DAG tells us which variables to include in the analysis, but it does not specify how to estimate the causal effect of interest. There are three key methods to estimate the causal effect: stratifying, matching, and weighting. The following subsections describe each of these in turn.

8.5.1 *Stratifying*

A stratified analysis calculates the causal effect at each level of the confounding variables. Since all non-causal paths are blocked, any difference in outcomes between individuals is attributed to the causal variable X or to random noise. In fact, we can think of each stratum as a controlled experiment that randomly assigned individuals to different treatment groups of X, so that these groups are comparable and the causal effect is estimated in each stratum using a simple difference in means.

For example, consider again the kidney stone example represented as a DAG in Fig. 8.5. For D-separation, we need to control for stone size, a variable that has two levels, small and large. A stratified analysis calculates the effect in each stratum separately. From Table 8.1, the raw success rates for patients who had small stones were 93.1% for open surgery and 86.7% for PCNL. For large stones, the raw success rates were 73.0% and 68.8%, respectively. The differences in raw success rates in the two strata were thus 6.4% and 4.2%. These are stratum-specific causal effects.

To estimate the overall causal effect, we need to account for the proportions of patients in the two strata in the population of interest. The causal effect can be calculated using a weighted average of success rates across the strata, with weights reflecting the composition of the population. A standard approach is to use the composition in the sample as reflecting that in the population. In the current example, 51% of patients had small stones and 49% had large stones, so a weighted average gives a success rate of $0.51 \times 93.1\% + 0.49 \times 73.0\% = 83.3\%$ for open

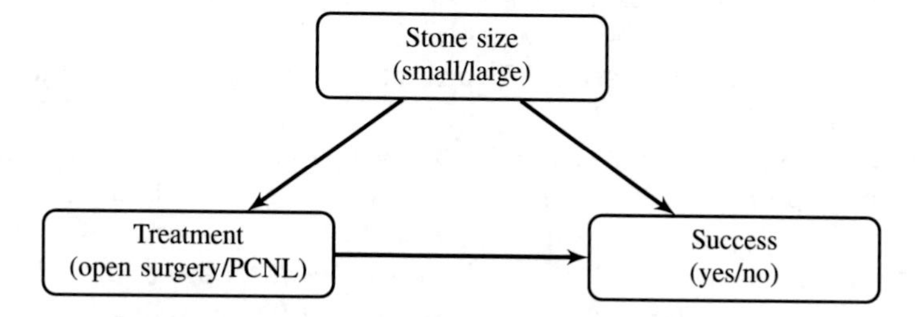

Fig. 8.5 Causal graph for treatment of kidney stones

surgery and $0.51 \times 86.7\% + 0.49 \times 68.8\% = 77.9\%$ for PCNL. The causal effect is therefore $83.3\% - 77.9\% = 5.4\%$. This means that about 5.4% more successes are expected if all patients are treated with open surgery compared to if all patients are treated with PCNL in a population comprising 51% patients with small stones and 49% patients with large stones.

Whether to report stratum-specific effects or an overall causal effect (and what weights to use) depends on the scientific question, but a critical assumption for any causal inference is that all non-causal paths are captured in the DAG and properly accounted for by the stratification.

What if achieving D-separation requires us to stratify on several variables? In that case, the strata are defined by the factorial combination of the levels of all stratifying variables, and the number of strata can become quite large. The number of strata also becomes large when there is a continuous confounder. In such cases, we might make additional assumptions about the structure of the effect. One approach is to define coarser strata by some measure of similarity between individuals, so, for example, subjects of similar ages (say within the same 5-year age group) can form one stratum.

Another common approach to handle several stratification variables at once is by fitting a linear regression model that includes these variables. This amounts to assuming that a linear regression model holds (see Chap. 3) and specifically that a change in the level of the cause implies a change in the outcome that is similar across all combinations of stratifying variables. The estimated effect is given by the coefficient of the cause variable X in the regression model. In the kidney stone example, a similar estimate of the causal effect (5.3%) is obtained from the coefficient for treatment in a linear regression fit to the proportion of successes and controlling for kidney size.

For an example involving several stratification variables, we use the 2017 sample data from Medical Expenditure Panel Survey (MEPS). MEPS is a rolling panel survey of health conditions, medical costs, and participant socio-demographics from thousands of persons in the United States. It has been continuously fielded since 1996 [10].

We use the MEPS data to study the effect of arthritis on health expenditures based on the causal graph in Fig. 8.4. Since a fraction of the population has no health expenditures during the year, we develop a causal two-part model for health expenditures as discussed in Chap. 6. Thus, we fit one model where the outcome is an indicator of any health expenditures during the year, and we fit another model for the amount among persons with non-zero expenditures. We use data only on individuals age 18 years or older and for presentation purposes remove observations with missing data on any variables.

The second and third columns of Table 8.2 show results of the logistic regression for having any positive health expenditures versus having none. The estimated effect of arthritis is 1.21, which means that the odds of positive expenditures for persons with arthritis are about $\exp(1.21) = 3.37$ times the odds for those who do not have arthritis, with 95% confidence interval $\exp(1.21 \pm 1.96 \times 0.08) = (2.87, 3.92)$. As always, the validity of these results depends on the validity of our modeling

Table 8.2 Two-part model of effects of arthritis on health expenditures based on MEPS 2017 sample data: logistic regression for effect on any health expenditures and linear regression for the amount of health expenditures among persons with non-zero health expenditures

Variable	Coef. (logistic)	SE (logistic)	Coef. (linear)	SE (linear)
Intercept	−0.40	0.06	224.56	467.51
Arthritis = yes	1.21	0.08	4106.62	343.06
Sex = female	0.80	0.04	407.30	286.15
Diabetes = yes	1.72	0.14	6052.36	413.54
Age	0.03	0.00	97.27	8.93

assumptions, which are compromised if important confounders are missing or the regression model is mis-specified.

The fourth and fifth columns of Table 8.2 show the results of the linear regression for the amount of health expenditures among persons who had non-zero expenditures. In this subpopulation, the mean health expenditures for those with arthritis were \$4106.62 higher than those without, with 95% confidence interval $\$4106.62 \pm 1.96 \times 343.06 = (\$3434.22, \$4779.02)$. As before, this greater health expenditure applies for any combination of age, sex, and diabetes status because the model is linear and has no interactions. We conclude that having arthritis not only increases the probability of having health expenditures; it also increases the amount of health expenditures.

The linear model has a causal interpretation only when restricting the population to patients having some expenditures during the year. This sub-population is not defined at the beginning of the year, and, therefore, interpretation of this part is problematic. However, it can be combined with the first part (the logistic regression) to calculate the total effect of arthritis by scaling the predicted amount of health expenditures from the second model by the predicted probability of having health expenditures from the first model. Doing this calculation as if all persons in the sample data had arthritis yields a mean health expenditure of \$9440, and repeating this calculation as if no persons in the sample data had arthritis yields a mean health expenditure of \$5084, so the average causal effect is estimated to be \$4356. Interestingly, calculating simple means among persons with and without arthritis, and therefore ignoring confounding, yields mean health expenditures of \$11,666 and \$4299, respectively, or a difference of \$7367, which is substantially higher than the estimate obtained when controlling for confounders.

The foregoing analysis mainly serves for illustration. A more complete analysis would examine other potential confounders, consider transformations and/or interactions, more appropriately account for missing data, and account for survey sampling weights. These issues show how challenging it can be to learn from observational data and how careful and knowledgeable the researcher should be in order to obtain valid and meaningful results.

8.5.2 Matching

A matched analysis aims to correct for selection by creating comparable distributions of confounders at each level of the causal variable X. This idea is easiest to illustrate for a binary causal variable X, such as kidney stone treatment (open surgery/PCNL) or arthritis (yes/no). To assess the causal effect of a binary variable X on the outcome Y, each subject with $X = 0$ is matched to a subject with $X = 1$ who has the same values of all the confounders. This leads to a structure similar to a randomized experiment, where the causal effect is estimated as the difference in mean outcomes between the two groups, possibly using weights to account for differences in population structure. Thus, whereas the stratification approach adjusts the analysis for confounding, the matching approach adjusts the data.

Applying this method to the kidney stone example, we match subjects in the two treatment groups according to stone size. Specifically, to match the 87 patients in the small-stone open surgery group, we randomly select 87 of the 270 patients in the small-stone PCNL group. Similarly, to match the 80 patients from the large-stone PCNL group, we randomly select 80 of the 263 patients in the large-stone open surgery group. Repeating this random sampling step 100 times (to reduce the sampling error), we calculate mean success rates of 82.8% in the open surgery group and 77.7% in the PCNL group. The simple difference of 5.1% between treatment groups is the estimated causal effect for a population having a ratio of 87:80 of small versus large stones.

Returning to the arthritis example, there are three covariates that should be matched on: age, sex, and diabetes. For each individual with arthritis, it can be difficult or impossible to find an individual without arthritis having exactly the same values for age, sex, and diabetes status. In such cases, we can replace exact matching with approximate matching for some variables. For example, we can match exactly on the binary variables sex and diabetes but allow for ages to slightly deviate up to a specified range.

Matching can be challenging computationally, but fortunately there are functions that do the work for us [11, 12]. For this example, we match exactly on sex and diabetes and use a nearest-neighbor matching algorithm to match on age, allowing deviations of up to 10 years. The *nearest-neighbor* algorithm is just one of several methods to select matches; as its name suggests, it identifies the closest available match. The procedure successfully matches 4749 of the 5309 persons with arthritis to persons without arthritis in the MEPS 2017 sample data. Using these 4749 matched pairs, mean health expenditures are $11,136 and $6528 in the arthritis and no-arthritis groups, respectively, a difference of $4608. This estimated effect is for a population with a distribution of the confounding variables as observed in the matched data, which may differ from the overall population. As mentioned above, different weighted averages can give the average effect for populations with different distributions of the confounders.

Matching can be done not only in a 1:1 ratio but also in a 1:m ratio (for some $m > 1$), and also when there are more than two groups. The key is to achieve a distribution of the confounding variables that is similar at each level of the causal variable X. One can also use stratification after matching if estimating the effects in sub-groups is of interest or fit a regression model to the matched data to improve precision. A review of matching methods and practical recommendations can be found in Stuart [11].

8.5.3 Weighting

The weighting approach links directly to the notion of selection, and specifically to the likelihood of individuals selecting different values of the cause variable based on their values of the confounding variables. In the kidney stone example, the chance of selecting open surgery was higher for individuals with larger stones, and the chance of selecting PCNL was higher for individuals with smaller stones. Thus, individuals with different values for the confounding variables had different chances of selecting one treatment versus another. Weighting is designed to restore the sample to one in which the confounders do not affect treatment selection. When we use this method, we weight each individual in the sample to create a pseudo-population in which an individual has the same chance of selecting each treatment regardless of their values of the confounding variables. Outcomes within each pseudo-population are then compared directly as if they were obtained in a randomized trial.

When we think about randomized trials, we usually imagine flipping a fair coin that determines the treatment or control assignment for each subject. In this case, the probability of assignment to each group is $1/2$; the trial perfectly reflects a population in which individuals have the same chance of selecting each treatment regardless of their characteristics. What if the coin is not fair, and it assigns a case to an experimental treatment with probability $1/4$ and to the control group with probability $3/4$? Then, on average, out of four enrolled participants, only one goes to the treatment group, and three go to the control group. As a consequence, the control group will have three times as many participants as the experimental treatment group. To generate a pseudo-population that remedies this imbalance requires upweighting the outcomes in the treatment group relative to the control group. Weighting the outcomes in the treatment group by 4 and in the control group by $4/3$ yields the desired result. In general, if an individual has a probability π of assignment to a treatment group, his/her outcomes should be weighted by $1/\pi$ to construct the desired pseudo-population in which treatment and control assignment are independent of confounders.

The method of weighting has been used for many years in survey sampling, where the well-known Horvitz–Thompson estimator for the mean of a variable Y in the population uses weighting to accommodate differential sampling probabilities. The Horvitz–Thompson estimator is given by the weighted average:

$$\text{Estimated mean of } Y = \frac{\sum_{i=1}^{n} w_i Y_i}{\sum_{i=1}^{n} w_i},$$

where $w_i = 1/\pi_i$ is the reciprocal of the probability that subject i is included in the sample of n subjects. Informally, if the probability π_i is not equal to 0 or 1 for all individuals, the numerator $\sum_{i=1}^{n} w_i Y_i$ estimates the population total of Y, and the denominator $\sum_{i=1}^{n} w_i$ estimates the population size.

In observational studies, suppose that a subject with confounder Z has probability $\pi(Z)$ of selecting treatment $X = 1$, that is, $P(X = 1 \mid Z) = \pi(Z)$, and the complement probability of being in the control group, $P(X = 0 \mid Z) = 1 - \pi(Z)$. If every subject is eligible for either treatment, so that $\pi(Z) \neq 0$ and $\pi(Z) \neq 1$, then an unbiased estimate of the causal effect is given by:

$$\text{Causal effect} = \frac{\sum_{i \in A} Y_i/\pi(Z_i)}{\sum_{i \in A} 1/\pi(Z_i)} - \frac{\sum_{j \in B} Y_j/(1 - \pi(Z_j))}{\sum_{j \in B} 1/(1 - \pi(Z_j))},$$

where A and B index the participants selecting treatment $X = 1$ and $X = 0$, respectively. This equation tells us to calculate weighted averages in the treatment and control groups and then take the difference. In the treatment group, the weights are given by the inverse of the probability of selecting into the treatment group, and in the control group, the weights are given by the inverse of the probability of selecting into the control group. The confounders determine these probabilities for the two groups. Because these differential selection probabilities induce selection bias, in principle, the inverse weighting should correct for this bias. However, it is not always clear how to calculate the selection probabilities, and assuming a specific functional form for $\pi(Z)$ adds a new possibility of model mis-specification.

We demonstrate the weighting method using the kidney stone example. First, we estimate the probability of a patient selecting each treatment according to stone size using the observed proportions. The estimated probabilities of patients with small and large stones selecting open surgery are:

$$P(\text{open surgery} \mid \text{small}) = 87/357$$
$$P(\text{open surgery} \mid \text{large}) = 263/343.$$

Therefore, the 81 successful open surgeries for patients with small stones should be upweighted to $81/(87/357) = 332.4$ successes out of $87/(87/357) = 357$ patients with small stones in the pseudo-population. Similarly, the 192 successes of open surgeries for patients having large stones represent $192/(263/343) = 250.4$ successes among a total of $263/(263/343) = 343$ patients with large stones in the pseudo-population. Thus, in the pseudo-population of $357+343 = 700$ patients who received open surgery, $332.4 + 250.4 = 582.8$ or 83.3% were successful. Similar calculations for PCNL give a success rate of 77.9%, so the estimated causal effect is $83.3\% - 77.9\% = 5.4\%$. This is the same result as the stratified analysis; the weighting and stratifying approaches are equivalent when the weights are calculated from the observed strata. However, when weights are calculated by other means, as discussed in the next section, the two approaches differ.

8.6 Propensity Scores

Many scientific questions involve large numbers of confounders, making stratifying, matching, or weighting challenging to implement. Propensity score analysis is a way to balance assignment to the cause variable X in this setting. The method involves two steps. First, we estimate propensity scores, which combine information on all the confounders. Second, we use the propensity scores as a basis for stratifying, matching, or weighting.

The idea of the propensity score was formally introduced by Rosenbaum and Rubin [13]. The propensity score, $\pi(Z)$, is the probability of selecting treatment group $X = 1$ given confounders Z. In the kidney stone example discussed in the previous subsection, where there was only one confounder ($Z =$ stone size), we calculated a propensity score as the probability of each treatment conditional on Z. When there are many confounders, the propensity score $\pi(Z)$ captures the joint impact of them all on treatment selection in a single metric.

A key result is that under two conditions—(1) the treatment assignment mechanism is a function *only* of observed covariates (i.e., all elements of Z are observed) and (2) all individuals studied are eligible for all treatments—the propensity score is a balancing score. In other words, under these conditions, conditional on the propensity score, the treatment status X is independent of the confounding variables. This is a striking result because it means that, if conditions (1) and (2) are satisfied, a treated subject and a control subject with exactly the same value of $\pi(Z)$ are comparable even if their values of the confounders are very different, e.g., one can be an 80-year-old male and the other a 20-year-old female. As long as the propensity score is the same, these subjects can be compared without worrying about confounding. This means that, once propensity scores are calculated for all individuals, the analysis can be conducted via any of the methods described above [13]. We can stratify by propensity score values, either dividing the scores into K strata or controlling the scores via regression analysis. We can match individuals according to their propensity scores and simply compare the mean outcomes in the matched samples. Or we can do a weighted comparison using the inverse of the propensity score for an individual's assigned treatment group as his/her weight.

The standard method for estimating propensity scores is to fit a regression model in which the outcome is an indicator of the treatment group and the covariates are the confounding variables. If the treatment is binary, logistic regression is traditionally used (see Chap. 4). More recently, and when the number of confounders is very large, machine learning approaches are being explored for propensity score estimation [14, 15].

We demonstrate propensity score estimation and analysis via stratifying, matching, and weighting using the arthritis example. First, we fit a logistic regression to

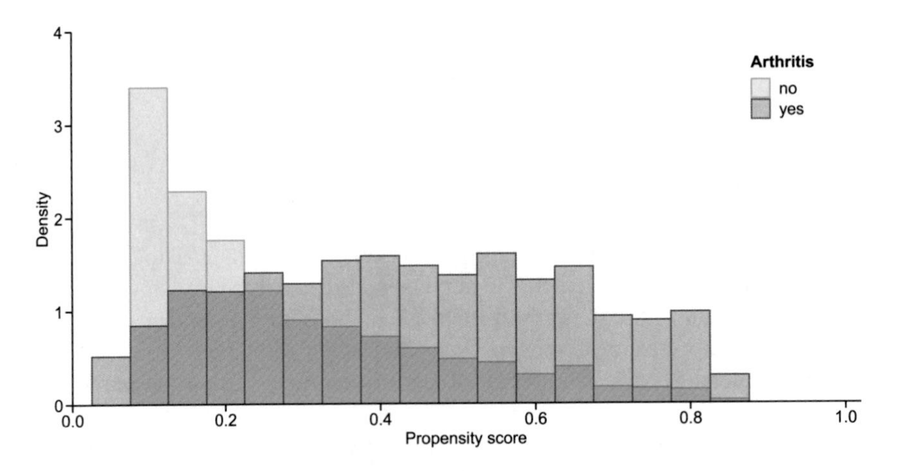

Fig. 8.6 Histograms of propensity scores by arthritis status

Table 8.3 Difference in average health expenditures between persons with and without arthritis from MEPS 2017 sample data based on unconditional analysis and propensity score analyses with stratifying, matching, and weighting

Method	Cost (no arthritis)	Cost (arthritis)	Cost difference
No conditioning	$4299	$11,666	$7367
Stratifying	$5126	$9961	$4835
Matching	$6528	$11,136	$4608
Weighting	$5290	$10,153	$4863

estimate arthritis status based on age, sex, and diabetes. The propensity scores are given by the fitted probabilities (Fig. 8.6). The stratifying analysis calculates the stratum-specific mean difference of total expenditures between those who do and those who do not have arthritis and then averages the results across the strata using the stratum sizes as weights. The matching analysis is identical to that described in Sect. 8.5.2, where observations are matched by nearest-neighbor matching on the propensity scores. The weighting analysis calculates weights using the inverse propensity score in the arthritis group and the inverse of one minus the propensity score in the no-arthritis group. Then, it calculates the weighted mean of total expenditures in each group and estimates the average causal effect by the difference between the weighted means. Results are shown in Table 8.3.

Table 8.3 shows average health expenditures in arthritis and no-arthritis groups and the causal estimate of the difference in expenditures. Results of an unconditional analysis are shown for comparison. Note that the unconditional analysis is unadjusted and should not be interpreted as a causal effect. In contrast, the propensity score analyses estimate the causal effect of arthritis on health expenditures so long as the two key assumptions for propensity score analysis are satisfied and the propensity score model is not mis-specified.

The relative merits of stratifying, matching, and weighting have been discussed extensively; see Austin [16] for a review and Lunceford and Davidian [17] for a comparison of stratifying and matching in terms of their balancing properties. Although, in principle, regression adjustment (i.e., including the propensity score as a covariate in a regression of the outcome on the treatment variable) might appear to be a reasonable way of stratifying, it is not a preferred approach because it does not control for selection bias as well as the other approaches [18]. As we have already observed, matching is straightforward in principle, but it can lead to a significant reduction in the data used for analysis. The three approaches can be biased if the model for the propensity score is missing important confounders or if it is mis-specified. To account for the latter problem, Funk et al. [19] discuss a doubly robust approach that uses both stratification and weighting. It is based on two regressions, one for the propensity score and one for the outcome, and produces results that are robust to mis-specification of either of these models, although not both. The doubly robust approach has received a great deal of attention in the statistical literature as part of a continuing evolution of the methodological base for causal inference using propensity score models.

8.7 Mediation Analysis

In causal analysis, questions often arise about the mechanism driving an observed causal effect—what variables are involved in the process and what is the contribution of each? This is exactly the goal of mediation analysis. The variables Z in the causal path from X to Y that explain the effect of X on Y are called *mediators*. These variables are not used for calculation of the causal effect but are important when we want to break it down into its components.

In the arthritis example, a key question concerns the role of pain in explaining the increased medical expenditures associated with arthritis. To what extent is the increment in expenditures driven by the effect of arthritis on chronic pain? To address this question, we explore the two causal paths depicted in blue in Fig. 8.4: the direct path from arthritis to health expenditures and the indirect path mediated through pain. The results of such an analysis can guide us in making important medical decisions. For example, if the effect along the indirect path is substantially greater than the effect along the direct path, so that much of the incremental health expenditures due to arthritis are mediated by pain, we might prioritize pain-reducing treatments for arthritis over other interventions to reduce these costs.

Mediation analysis is simplest when both the outcome variable (here, health expenditures) and the mediator (here, pain) are both continuous, and a linear model can be used. We focus here on individuals who had non-zero health expenditures, and, for this sub-group, we study the contribution of pain to the increase in costs. Pain is an ordinal variable in MEPS measured on a scale from 1 to 5, and an alternative model might consider pain as such or as a binary variable after combining

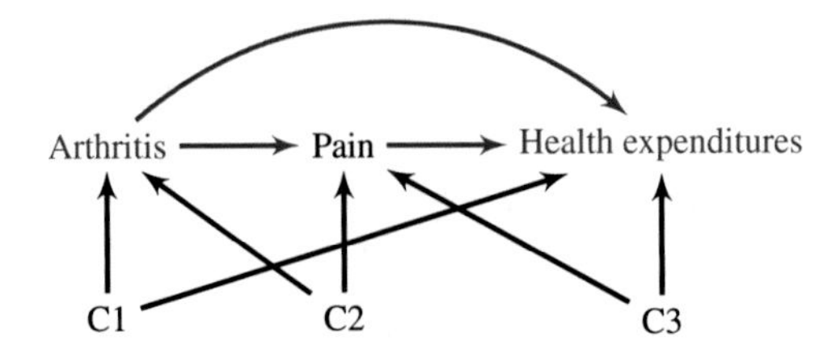

Fig. 8.7 Pain as a mediator of the effect of arthritis on health expenditures. The variables C1, C2, and C3 are confounders for three causal models: (1) health expenditures given arthritis, (2) pain given arthritis, and (3) health expenditures given pain, respectively

categories. However, to demonstrate the method, we assume simple linear models. For mediation analysis under more complex models, see VanderWeele [20, 21].

Figure 8.7 presents the DAG for this mediation analysis. The total effect of arthritis on health expenditures is the combined effect of the direct and indirect causal paths. The mediation analysis partitions the total effect into the direct effect and the indirect effect.

There are three causal models that are relevant: (1) health expenditures (outcome) given arthritis (cause), (2) pain (outcome) given arthritis (cause), and (3) health expenditures (outcome) given pain (cause). The first model estimates the total effect; models (2) and (3) estimate the indirect effect. We denote the confounding variables for these models C1, C2, and C3. C1 is the set of confounders for the effect of arthritis on health expenditures, C2 is the set of confounders for the effect of arthritis on pain, and C3 is the set of confounders for the effect of pain on health expenditures. In our example, the confounders for all three models were age, sex, and diabetes. The mediation analysis fits three regression models; each model must include the full set of confounding variables C1, C2, and C3. In addition, model (3) includes arthritis as a covariate because, based on the DAG, arthritis is a confounder of the pain–expenditures pathway.

Table 8.4 shows the three linear regression models. Note the coefficients for the cause variable in each model. In model (1), the estimated coefficient \$4106.62 is the total effect of arthritis on expenditures. In model (2), 0.82 is the effect of arthritis on pain, and, in model (3), \$3172.94 is the effect of pain on medical expenditures. The estimate of 0.82 in model (2) means that arthritis increases pain by 0.82 "pain units"; the \$3172.94 in model (3) means that a "one unit" increase in pain translates into a \$3172.94 increase in health expenditures, so the estimated indirect effect of arthritis is $0.82 \times \$3172.94 = \$2610.88$. The direct effect is then the difference between the total effect and the indirect effect: $\$4106.62 - \$2610.88 = \$1495.74$.

When the three models are linear, the above estimate of the direct effect, which was popularized by Baron and Kenny [22], coincides with the coefficient of arthritis in model (3), and the indirect effect can be obtained as the difference between the coefficients of arthritis in models (1) and (3) (so fitting model (2) is not required for mediation analysis). In the jargon of causal inference, including pain in model (3) *blocks* the path:

Table 8.4 Fitted regression models in the mediation analysis of the effect of arthritis on health expenditures using the MEPS 2017 sample data

Variable	Coef. (1)	SE (1)	Coef. (2)	SE (2)	Coef. (3)	SE (3)
Intercept	224.56	467.51	1.13	0.03	−3365.59	487.35
Arthritis = yes	4106.62	343.06	0.82	0.02	1495.74	357.28
Sex = female	407.30	286.15	0.06	0.02	206.35	282.04
Diabetes = yes	6052.36	413.54	0.41	0.02	4747.49	411.48
Age	97.27	8.93	0.01	0.00	78.35	8.84
Pain	–	–	–	–	3172.94	140.86

$$\text{arthritis} \rightarrow \text{pain} \rightarrow \text{health expenditures}$$

and leaves only the direct effect of arthritis on health expenditures. We would conclude that the effect of arthritis on health expenditures is largely mediated by pain, with around $1495.74/4106.62 = 36\%$ of the total effect attributable to the indirect effect of pain.

Complete mediation is defined as the presence of a significant indirect effect and a null direct effect. In practice, this characterization is identified via significance testing of the indirect effect and examination of the magnitude of the direct effect as expressed by the coefficient of X (arthritis) in a regression that also includes the mediator Z (pain). If this coefficient is zero or close to zero, then the effect of X on Y is said to be completely mediated by Z.

An essential assumption for mediation analysis is that there must be no causal path from arthritis to C3; that is, the cause variable should not affect the confounders of the association between the mediator and the outcome. If such an arrow exists, then C3 is also a mediator, and the analysis becomes more challenging [20, 21].

The process of mediation is inherently temporal. For X to affect Z, and for Z in turn to affect Y, there must be a sensible temporal relationship across the three variables, and the timing of measuring each should reflect this sequential relationship. Thus, mediation analysis may not be appropriate in all cross-sectional data settings [23]. In the arthritis example, determining the temporal relationships between the variables in the MEPS data takes some sleuthing. It turns out that medical condition indicators in MEPS reflect conditions ascertained at any time during the year, pain is reported in the survey conducted in the middle of the year, and health expenditures are cumulative over the year. Thus, a legitimate critique of this mediation analysis concerns the timing of the assessments of X, Y, and Z.

The basic framework of Baron and Kenny [22] has been closely scrutinized over the years. The framework was designed for linear models and must be modified when the mediator or outcome (or both) are binary or when the linear model assumptions do not hold. The approach does not accommodate moderated mediation, i.e., settings in which the mediation effect varies by the level of the cause variable X (arthritis)—that is, when there is an interaction between the cause variable and the mediator (between arthritis and pain). Moderated mediation may be a concern in the arthritis example if the effect of pain on medical costs differs among those with and without arthritis. Adding an interaction term to model (3) in Table 8.4 yields a non-significant result, suggesting that moderation may not be an issue in this analysis. When interactions are not ignorable, extensions to the direct and indirect effects have been suggested, but their calculation and, more importantly, their interpretation are not as simple as in the linear, non-interaction case. For a discussion of these issues, see VanderWeele and Vansteelandt [24], who defined these concepts in terms of potential outcomes, a framework that is discussed in the next section.

8.8 Potential Outcomes

So far, we have defined causality only informally as the mechanism that drives how the outcome changes in response to a change in the cause. Practically, we noted that the causal effect is the effect observed in large randomized clinical trials. However, the randomization does not generate the outcomes; it simply determines a framework for observing the outcomes. In contrast, causality is understood as a more basic mechanism that generates the outcomes.

The concept of potential outcomes formalizes the meaning of causality and enables the development of mathematical theory and statistical methods for estimation. No discussion of causality is complete without mentioning the concept, but we will not develop any mathematics here. There is vast literature on the topic (e.g., [25]).

Returning to the basic scientific problem, an individual causal effect is naturally defined as the answer to the following question: what would have happened to the outcome if an individual had been treated compared to if they had not been treated? (We use the term "treatment" to refer to a generic binary cause variable for the purpose of discussion.) This question, stated at the individual level, is exactly what most people imagine a causal effect to be. However, this question is hypothetical as the two possibilities (treated/not treated) cannot coexist. Nevertheless, we can define the outcomes of an individual in the two possible scenarios, calling them *potential outcomes* or *counterfactuals*.

To illustrate this idea, imagine that, prior to the outcome being observed, individual i could be assigned to each level of the treatment, $X = 0$ and $X = 1$, with two corresponding potential outcomes, denoted Y_{i0} and Y_{i1}. We can then imagine that the individual has two representations of his/her exposure and outcome values, $(0, Y_{i0})$ and $(1, Y_{i1})$. The causal effect for individual i is simply $Y_{i1} - Y_{i0}$, and the average causal effect is defined as $\text{ACE} = \overline{Y}_1 - \overline{Y}_0$, the average of the individual causal effects.

In practice, we can only observe one of $(0, Y_{i0})$ and $(1, Y_{i1})$, the former if the treatment allocation is $X = 0$ and the latter if it is $X = 1$. In randomized trials, by assigning X at random to treatment groups (0 or 1), we protect against the influence of other factors on the mechanism by which a potential outcome is realized for individual i, and this facilitates unbiased estimation of the ACE. In observational studies, the mechanism by which X and the corresponding potential outcome are realized for individual i can and usually does depend on other factors. DAGs enable us to identify which of these are confounders, and causal theory tells us that, so long as all confounders are observed, the methods developed in this chapter permit us to replicate the circumstances of randomized assignment in which treatment selection is independent of confounders. This, in turn, facilitates unbiased estimation of the ACE defined via potential outcomes.

8.9 Software and Data

R code to download data and to carry out the examples in this book is available at the GitHub page https://roman-gulati.github.io/statistics-for-health-data-science/. In addition to the R packages cited in Chap. 1, this chapter also used the `MatchIt` package [12].

References

1. Fisher, R.A.: Dangers of cigarette-smoking. Br. Med. J. **2**(5039), 297 (1957)
2. Charig, C.R., Webb, D.R., Payne, S.R., Wickham, J.E.: Comparison of treatment of renal calculi by open surgery, percutaneous nephrolithotomy, and extracorporeal shockwave lithotripsy. Br. Med. J. **292**(6524), 879–882 (1986)
3. Pearl, J., Mackenzie, D.: The Book of Why: The New Science of Cause and Effect. Basic Books, New York (2018)
4. Bickel, P.J., Hammel, E.A., O'Connell, J.W.: Sex bias in graduate admissions: Data from Berkeley. Science **187**(4175), 398–404 (1975)
5. Hancock, D.B., Guo, Y., Reginsson, G.W., Gaddis, N.C., Lutz, S.M., Sherva, R., Loukola, A., Minica, C.C., Markunas, C.A., Han, Y., et al.: Genome-wide association study across European and African American ancestries identifies a SNP in DNMT3B contributing to nicotine dependence. Mol. Psychiatry **23**(9), 1911–1919 (2018)
6. Berkson, J.: Limitations of the application of fourfold table analysis to hospital data. Biomet. Bull. **2**(3), 47–53 (1946)
7. van Vollenhoven, R.F.: Sex differences in rhematoid arthritis: more than meets the eye. BMC Med. **7**, 12 (2012)
8. Rehling, T., Bjorkman, A.D., Andersen, M.B., Ekholm, O., Molsted, S.: Diabetes is associated with musculoskeletal pain, osteoarthritis, osteoporosis, and rheumatoid arthritis. J. Diabetes Res. **2019**, 1–6 (2019)
9. Lederer, D.J., Bell, S.C., Branson, R.D., Chalmers, J.D., Marshall, R., Maslove, D.M., Ost, D.E., Punjabi, N.M., Schatz, M., Smyth, A.R., et al.: Control of confounding and reporting of results in causal inference studies. Guidance for authors from editors of respiratory, sleep, and critical care journals. Ann. Am. Thoracic Soc. **16**(1), 22–28 (2019)
10. For Healthcare Research, A., Quality: Medical expenditure panel survey (). http://www.ahrq.gov/research/data/meps/index.html. Accessed 12 Feb 2020
11. Stuart, E.A.: Matching methods for causal inference: a review and a look forward. Stat. Sci. **25**(1), 1 (2010)

12. Ho, D.E., Imai, K., King, G., Stuart, E.A., et al.: Matchit: nonparametric preprocessing for parametric causal inference. J. Stat. Softw. **42**(8), 1–28 (2011). http://www.jstatsoft.org/v42/i08/
13. Rosenbaum, P.R., Rubin, D.B.: The central role of the propensity score in observational studies for causal effects. Biometrika **70**(1), 41–55 (1983)
14. Nichols, A., McBride, L.: Propensity scores and causal inference using machine learning methods. In: 2017 Stata Conference 13. Stata Users Group (2017)
15. Westreich, D., Lessler, J., Funk, M.J.: Propensity score estimation: machine learning and classification methods as alternatives to logistic regression. J. Clin. Epidemiol. **63**, 826–833 (2010)
16. Austin, P.C.: An introduction to propensity score methods for reducing the effects of confounding in observational studies. Multivar. Behav. Res. **46**, 399–424 (2011)
17. Lunceford, J.K., Davidian, M.: Stratification and weighting via the propensity score in estimation of causal treatment effects. Stat. Med. **23**, 2937–2960 (2004)
18. Garrido, M.M.: Covariate adjustment and propensity scores. J. Am. Med. Assoc. **315**, 1521–1522 (2016)
19. Funk, M.J., Westreich, D., Wiesen, C., Sturmer, T., Brookhart, M.A., Davidian, M.: Doubly robust estimation of causal effects. Am. J. Epidemiol. **173**, 761–767 (2011)
20. VanderWeele, T.: Explanation in Causal Inference: Methods for Mediation and Interaction. Oxford University Press, Oxford (2015)
21. VanderWeele, T.J.: Mediation analysis: a practitioner's guide. Ann. Rev. Public Health **37**, 17–32 (2016)
22. Baron, R.M., Kenny, D.A.: The moderator-mediator variable distinction in social psychological research: conceptual, strategic, and statistical considerations. J. Pers. Soc. Psychol. **51**(6), 1173 (1986)
23. Maxwell, S.E., Cole, D.A.: Bias in cross-sectional analyses of longitudinal mediation. Psychol. Methods **12**, 23–34 (2007)
24. VanderWeele, T.J., Vansteelandt, S.: Conceptual issues concerning mediation, interventions and composition. Stat. Interface **2**(4), 457–468 (2009)
25. Hernán, M.A., Robins, J.M.: Causal inference: What if. Chapman & Hall/CRC, Boca Raton (2020)

Chapter 9
Survey Data Analysis

Abstract In previous chapters, we discussed the notions of samples and populations. After defining the population of interest, we drew a sample and used the sample estimates to make inferences about the population. In doing so, we acknowledged the importance of uncertainty and presented approaches to measure the variability in our estimates. Until now, we treated the samples as simple random samples, meaning that we assumed that subjects were drawn independently and with equal probability for every individual in the population. In this chapter, we study methods for analyzing data from health surveys, which rarely constitute simple random samples. Health surveys are a valuable tool for learning about population health and its correlates based on respondent self-report. After discussing key issues and concerns with self-reported data, we review several national health surveys in the United States. Most of the chapter focuses on survey data analysis and its dependence on the survey design. Key elements of survey design—stratification, clustering, and weighting—are described in detail. To demonstrate how to analyze a complex survey, we use data from the Medical Expenditure Panel Survey to estimate the annual expenditures associated with a prior diagnosis of diabetes in the US population.

9.1 Introduction

On December 1, 2015, *The New York Times* ran a triumphant headline, "New diabetes cases, at long last, begin to fall in the United States." The article referenced a report by the Centers for Disease Control and Prevention [1] that cited the number of new cases in the United States each year declining from approximately 1.7 million in 2009 to 1.4 million in 2014. The source of the data? The National Health Interview Survey [2].

The National Health Interview Survey (NHIS) is the largest in-person household survey in the United States. Conducted annually by the Census Bureau on behalf of the National Center for Health Statistics, the survey tracks the health of the US population, including the incidence and prevalence of a variety of health conditions. For the diabetes question, adult respondents were asked whether a health

R. Etzioni et al., *Statistics for Health Data Science*, Springer Texts in Statistics,
https://doi.org/10.1007/978-3-030-59889-1_9

professional had ever told them they had diabetes and if so their age at diagnosis. They were also asked their current age, allowing calculation of the interval from diagnosis to the survey, on the basis of which new diagnoses were identified.

Given the number of new diabetes cases in the survey data, how was it possible to produce the estimated number in the population? How reliable are such estimates and how can we quantify their uncertainty? This chapter addresses these questions.

9.2 Introduction to Health Surveys

Health surveys record individual responses to sets of questions designed to learn about a wide range of correlates of population health. These correlates may include sociodemographic and socioeconomic factors, health behaviors and conditions, access to health care, and individuals' perceptions of their health and their care. Health surveys are of enormous value because they directly query respondents for information that may be difficult or impossible to obtain from other sources, such as administrative data (see Chap. 1). At the same time, surveys are subject to a host of potential biases stemming from the very nature of self-reported information. Well-known potential biases associated with health surveys include non-response bias, recall bias, and social desirability bias.

Non-response bias arises when not all sampled subjects complete the survey—and those who do differ systematically from those who do not. In surveys that query individuals about their level of satisfaction, those who are dissatisfied are often more likely to respond than those who have no complaints. Another classic example of non-response bias occurs in the setting where patients are interviewed when they come for clinic visits, so only patients who are well enough to be seen in the clinic are able to respond. The possibility of non-response bias should be anticipated at the time of survey planning so that the mode and logistics of survey deployment can be devised accordingly. In the past, most large surveys were done by telephone or mail; now many surveys are conducted online. Each mode of survey deployment is subject to unique reasons for and mechanisms of non-response bias. In practice, most voluntary surveys are subject to some degree of non-response. Approaches for addressing missing data can be applied at the analysis stage, but these work best when the likelihood of non-response depends on known or observed factors, a type of missingness sometimes termed *missing at random*.

Recall bias occurs when participants cannot accurately remember past events—and their ability to do so is linked with the outcome of interest. For example, in a survey of factors explaining rates of cancer recurrence, cases that have recurred may have better recall of their initial treatments and complications than those who are recurrence-free. Mechanisms underlying recall bias have been extensively studied. Some of these can be addressed when planning the survey and designing survey questions.

Social desirability bias occurs when respondents are queried about behaviors that may be sensitive or known to be subject to disapproval, motivating them to respond in a certain way. Social desirability bias can be present when asking about alcohol use, dietary habits, and preventive behaviors, like wearing seatbelts or wearing face masks during a pandemic. Social desirability issues may also affect survey non-response.

Mitigation of these biases requires extensively researching and validating survey questions and carefully considering how potential biases might be impacted by the mode of survey implementation. Thus, even before the survey is deployed, a great deal of work must be done to develop the survey instrument, plan the logistics of survey deployment, and ensure that data infrastructure and processes for preserving confidentiality and ensuring that data quality are reliable.

In the rest of this chapter, we pick up after the survey has been conducted, when we have data from a survey sample and want to use it to learn about the underlying population. In previous chapters, we focused on estimating summaries of the population distribution of an outcome, such as the mean or median, and the association between these summaries and covariates. With population surveys, another objective emerges—to estimate population totals, such as the total number of individuals with a condition or the total incremental expenditures at the population level for that condition. We have already shown an example of the use of NHIS data to estimate the total number of newly diagnosed diabetes cases in the United States each year. The National Health and Nutrition Examination Survey (NHANES) data are the primary source of information on the prevalence of obesity in the population and how it is changing over time. And data from the Medical Expenditure Panel Survey (MEPS) can be used to project the total number of individuals with chronic pain in the United States and the associated annual health expenditures.

We will discuss the design of complex surveys and explain how the design affects the analysis and results. Very few large surveys use simple random samples because this design is neither as efficient nor as cost-effective as other methods. National surveys use multistage sampling, which involve stratification, clustering, and differential probabilities of selection. Differential probabilities of being sampled are reflected in weights attached to each sampled observation. We will show how to account for the survey design when calculating standard errors for survey-based estimates and how to use survey weights to scale up and produce population estimates of numbers of individuals affected by a condition and the attributable annual health expenditures, using a prior diabetes diagnosis as an example. First we briefly review three long-standing national health surveys in the United States as concrete examples of the principles and methods covered in this chapter.

9.3 National Health Surveys

The *National Health Interview Survey* (NHIS) [2] is the nation's largest in-person household health survey. Since 1957, the NHIS has been conducted annually by the Census Bureau on behalf of the National Center for Health Statistics (NCHS). The survey is cross-sectional and collects information on a different sample every year.

The NHIS questions cover a wide variety of topics, including medical conditions, health insurance, doctor visits, and health behaviors. Results from the NHIS have been used to monitor trends in the burden of chronic conditions and health care access and to track progress toward national health objectives.

The *National Health and Nutrition Examination Survey* (NHANES) [3], also conducted by the NCHS, goes one step further than the NHIS in that it not only interviews participants but also includes a full physical examination and blood test. While this step is logistically complex and adds significant cost, it yields objective measurements of important health indicators, such as blood pressure, body mass index, and hemoglobin A1c. NHANES data have been crucial in providing the data to create growth charts for children, monitor the prevalence of obese and overweight persons, and estimate the frequency of undiagnosed diabetes in the United States. National policies to eliminate lead in gasoline and food resources grew out of NHANES results. Similarly, ongoing national programs to reduce hypertension and cholesterol levels depend on NHANES data to target education and prevention efforts.

The *Medical Expenditure Panel Survey* (MEPS) [4], conducted by the Agency for Healthcare Research and Quality, collects extensive information on health care utilization and expenditures for a subsample of NHIS households. In addition to key sociodemographic, health history, and health behavior variables from the NHIS, the MEPS also includes detailed health insurance information as well as data on inpatient, outpatient, and prescription drug utilization, along with the corresponding expenditures sourced from medical providers and health records. The MEPS is a rolling panel survey that enrolls participants annually and interviews them five times over a period of 2 years. Thus, in contrast to the NHIS and NHANES, which are cross-sectional, the MEPS provides longitudinal information for a limited duration on each participant. MEPS data have been useful in tracking health care expenditures, identifying the most costly medical conditions, and monitoring the use of and costs of different types of care in the population.

9.4 Basic Elements of Survey Design

A survey is a probability sample; each unit in the population has a non-zero probability of being selected. The *sampling frame* is the master list of the units eligible for selection. In *simple random sampling*, every unit in the sampling frame has the same probability of being included. Most large population surveys do not use simple random sampling; they use stratification and clustering.

Stratified random sampling divides the population into predetermined subgroups, called *strata*, and samples independently from each stratum. Stratification is done to control the composition of the survey sample, and we will show that it can reduce the standard errors of survey-based estimates compared with simple random sampling when there is homogeneity within strata and heterogeneity across strata.

Clustered random sampling is the random sampling of groups of units, or clusters, within the population. Clustering is usually done to improve efficiency and reduce cost, but we will show that clustering can increase the standard errors of survey-based estimates relative to simple random sampling.

To illustrate the differences between stratification and clustering, consider a survey of undergraduate university students that asks about the number of hours spent on coursework outside of the classroom each week. The survey designers don't want the results to be skewed toward the sciences or the humanities, so they partition the student body into majors and decide to sample a fixed fraction of students within each major (assume there are no double majors). In this example, major is a stratifying variable; the number of strata (majors) is fixed and known in advance, the students within the different majors constitute independent samples, and students are drawn from every stratum. Further, strata defined by major may yield outcomes about study habits that are more homogeneous than using a simple random sample of the same size.

Now suppose the survey designers are concerned about non-response and social desirability biases and they feel both will be minimized if the survey is done in person. To save time and stretch the survey budget, instead of randomly sampling individuals within each stratum, they decide to randomly sample classes within each stratum and interview students in each selected class. The classes are clusters, also referred to as *primary sampling units*. If all students within each class are interviewed, the design is called a *single-stage clustering* design. If a random sample of students is selected within each class, the design is called a *two-stage clustering* design.

Why might two-stage clustering be preferred over single-stage clustering? The answer has to do with the reality that students within a class are likely to provide fairly similar answers to the question of interest. Indeed, there may be little to learn about study habits among students in the same class after a few have been interviewed. Compared to single-stage clustering with the same sample size, two-stage clustering offers the opportunity to gather data from more classes.

This example demonstrates a key difference between stratification and clustering, beyond the differing reasons for incorporating each in the survey design. With stratification, the strata are known in advance, and sampling units will be drawn from each one, so all strata will be represented in the final sample. With clustering, the number of clusters may be known in advance but which ones will be selected is not known, and not all clusters will be represented in the final sample.

This example illustrates stratification and clustering, and it suggests why these elements might be considered when designing a survey. Indeed, all of the aforementioned national surveys use stratification and clustering in complex *multistage designs*.

There is a direct line from the survey design to the variability of survey-based estimates. What do we mean by variability in the context of survey data analysis? In Chap. 7, we defined variability in terms of the long-run behavior or fluctuation in an estimate of interest if the sampling could be repeated many times. In this chapter, we return to this concept of variability and think of an estimate's standard error as a measure of the variation in the estimate if the survey could be repeated many times in the same population. In the following sections, we examine stratification and clustering in greater depth and show how they can impact the standard errors of survey-based estimates.

9.5 Stratified Sampling

Stratification has two main objectives: (1) to control the sample composition and (2) to reduce variability in the results. A stratified design controls the composition of the survey sample by partitioning the population into strata and pre-specifying the sampling fraction within each stratum. In practice, full control of sample composition is not possible due to participant non-response. Reweighting methods such as *post-stratification* and *raking* can be used to adjust the sample composition to what was intended in the design. We discuss these techniques later in this section. A stratified design often reduces the variance of the sample because strata tend to be more homogeneous than the overall population; this is also discussed below.

Examples of stratification variables include geographic location or demographic characteristics, such as age, sex, or race/ethnicity. Stratification by geographic location ensures that low-population locations, such as rural areas, will be sampled. Stratification by race/ethnicity ensures that minority groups will be adequately represented in the data.

Beyond ensuring that low-frequency population subgroups are included in the sample, which would not be guaranteed with simple random sampling, a stratified design can set the stratum-specific sampling fractions so that these sub-populations are sampled at higher rates than higher-frequency subgroups. This ensures sufficient representation in the survey sample for reliable subgroup analyses. In the NHIS, for example, strata are geographic and, until 2016, the survey oversampled African Americans, Hispanics, and Asian Americans. In 2016, the design of the survey was changed to oversample individuals in the ten least populous states [5]. The 2015–2018 NHANES oversampled certain race groups, age–sex groups, and age–race–income groups. For instance, one of the oversampled groups was "Non-Hispanic white persons and persons of other races and ethnicities aged 0–11 years or 80 years and over."

9.5.1 *Stratified Designs and Variance*

Partitioning of the population into strata and pre-specifying fixed sampling fractions within each lead to a reduction in variability in comparison with simple random sampling. This reduction occurs when the strata are chosen in a manner that induces within-stratum homogeneity and between-sample heterogeneity. To see why this is so, it is helpful to recall the definition of variability as a summary of the fluctuations in estimates if the survey could be done many times in the same population.

To explain the idea, consider a survey of self-reported health status stratified by age. It is well known that self-reported health status declines with age. Thus, older individuals have lower self-reported health than younger individuals. According to the 2018 Census Bureau's American Community Survey [6], 32% of the US population is younger than 25, 39% fall between 25 and 54, and 29% are older than 54. Suppose we conduct a survey of 1000 individuals, sampling the same fraction within each of these age groups: we sample 320 individuals younger than age 25 years, 390 individuals age 25–54 years, and 290 individuals older than age 54 years.

Now, imagine doing this survey many times. Each time, we sample the same number from each age group. If we have 100% response rate, all of the surveys will have the same age composition. This uniformity and predictability yield a survey sample that is lower in variability than the equivalent simple random sampling scheme. Why? Because under simple random sampling, the number sampled from each age group will change with every repeated survey. Some surveys will end up randomly selecting more individuals from the youngest age group and will have a preponderance of higher measures of self-reported health; conversely, some will end up randomly selecting more from the oldest age group, and self-reported health will skew lower. On average, the simple random design will end up sampling similar fractions from each stratum as the stratified design, but there will be greater variability across individual samples.

Table 9.1 shows the average fraction within each age group under repeated simple random sampling or repeated age-stratified sampling of MEPS 2017 participants (based on 100 replicates of 1000 participants each). Because there is no variation across age-stratified samples by construction, there is clearly less variability compared to simple random sampling. Consequently, we expect lower variability in outcomes that are correlated with age. In this example, the effect is modest; we find that the proportion of persons who reported being in excellent health in the MEPS 2017 data was 0.34 (95% CI 0.31–0.36) using simple random sampling and 0.34 (95% CI 0.32–0.37) using age-stratified sampling.

Mathematically, the variance under a stratified design is equal to a weighted sum across strata of the within-stratum variances, the weight of each stratum being determined by its relative size. Each stratum is its own independent sub-population. With k strata, there are k sub-populations, and if those k sub-populations are defined in a manner that creates similarity within and dissimilarity between sub-populations,

Table 9.1 Proportions and 95% confidence intervals of MEPS 2017 participants in various age groups selected by repeated simple random sampling or repeated age-stratified sampling, based on 100 replicates of 1000 participants each

Age	Simple random sampling	Age-stratified sampling
<25	0.34 (0.31, 0.37)	0.34 (0.34, 0.35)
25–54	0.38 (0.35, 0.41)	0.38 (0.38, 0.39)
>54	0.28 (0.25, 0.30)	0.27 (0.27, 0.28)

then the stratified design should lead to estimates that have lower standard errors than estimates obtained from a simple random sample.

9.5.2 *Stratification and Weighting*

One major change in perspective that accompanies survey data analysis is that rather than considering a sample as being from a theoretically infinite population, we acknowledge that we are sampling from a finite population and our goal is to produce results that are representative of that population. While a simple random sample produces a population-representative sample, it may miss low-frequency population subgroups, and as we have noted, this is one motivating reason to use stratified sampling. On the other hand, stratified samples that oversample population subgroups are not representative of the original population. This is generally the case with complex surveys, and to account for that, we reconstruct the composition of the original population using survey weights.

Under a given survey design, every individual in the population has a probability of being sampled. In simple random sampling, this probability is n/N, where n is the survey sample size and N is the size of the population. In a stratified random sample, where simple random sampling is conducted within each stratum, the probability of an individual in stratum i being sampled is n_i/N_i, where n_i is the sample size in stratum i and N_i is the size of stratum i. When estimating summaries like means or totals, we calculate weighted versions of these statistics, where the weights are given by the inverse of the sampling probabilities. Each weight corresponds to the number of individuals in the original population represented by that sampled individual. Thus, if a stratum has $N_i = 400$ individuals and we sample $n_i = 4$ individuals, the probability of each one being sampled is $1/100$, and each of these 4 sample units represents 100 observations and therefore will have weight equal to 100. As the sampling fractions can vary across strata, so can the weights.

Korn and Graubard [7] discuss survey weighting using an example from the Maternal and Infant Health Survey in 1988. This survey defined strata based on maternal race and infant birthweight, and it oversampled black mothers and low-birthweight infants. Specifically, among black mothers whose babies weighed less than 1500 g, 1 out of 14 were sampled, yielding a survey weight of 14. Conversely, among non-black mothers whose babies weighed more than 2500 g, 1 out of 720 were sampled, yielding a survey weight of 720. When estimating population summaries, weights are necessary; unweighted estimates are generally biased.

In practice, sampling fractions generally never turn out according to plan because of non-response. *Post-stratification* is a method for adjusting the survey weights to accommodate the observed non-response. As an example, suppose that the probability of non-response in our survey of self-reported health depends only on age and that only 80% of the youngest age group responds. In other words, only 4 out of 5 individuals planned to be in that stratum were actually present in the survey sample. Post-stratification would upweight those respondents by a factor of $5/4$, so their actual weight would be their intended weight times 1.25. Thus, post-stratification upweights different strata by different factors depending on their specific non-response rates.

When there are multiple stratification variables, a post-stratification technique called *raking* is used to adjust the stratum-specific weights so that the weighted sample is representative of the distribution of each of the stratification variables, in a marginal sense. Thus, in the Maternal and Infant Health Survey, where there were six strata defined by combinations of maternal race (two categories) and infant birthweight (three categories), raking would yield weights calibrated so that the weighted sample was representative of the population in terms of both maternal race and infant birthweight.

There are two important takeaways regarding post-stratification. First, standard post-stratification methods that produce multiplicative factors for design-based sample weights assume that non-responding and responding individuals within a stratum are essentially interchangeable. Second, post-stratification multipliers are not known in advance; they can only be determined once the survey has been implemented. Consequently, post-stratification-based weights are random and data-based, and their variability must be incorporated when estimating standard errors. This complicates estimating standard errors considerably. We discuss different approaches for dealing with these complications later in this chapter. First, we turn to another key element of survey design which has its own ramifications for variability: clustering.

9.6 Clustered Sampling

In clustered sampling designs, groups of individuals (clusters) are sampled together for reasons of convenience and economy. Both the NHIS and NHANES are in-person surveys and must cluster individuals by location for feasibility reasons. Natural clusters include households, schools, hospitals, and counties.

In the same way that a simple random sample draws from a sampling frame or list of eligible individuals, a clustered sample draws from a list of clusters. In a single-stage sample, all individuals in selected clusters are interviewed; in a two-stage sample, individuals are randomly drawn from within each selected cluster to be interviewed.

Figure 9.1 shows schematic illustrations of stratified and one- and two-stage clustered designs modeled after a similar figure in Lohr [8]. The figure also illustrates the differences between stratification and clustering. Strata are known and constitute an exhaustive partitioning of the population. The sample draws with certainty from each stratum based on pre-specified sampling fractions. Because the strata are known in advance, there is no randomness in the selection of strata. The only variability comes from the within-stratum variances.

Clusters are also specified in advance, but the sample does not draw with certainty from each cluster. Instead, only some clusters are sampled, and which

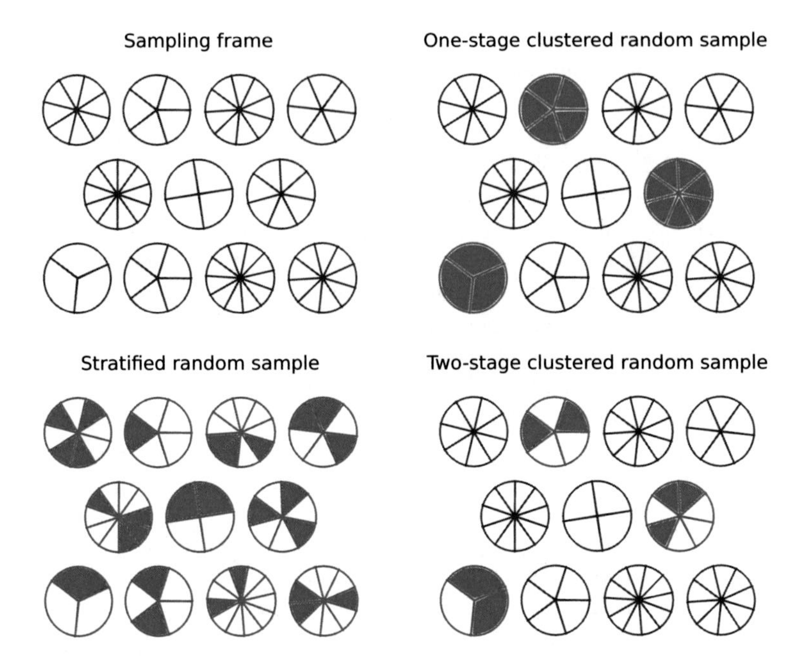

Fig. 9.1 Schematic illustrations of stratified random sampling and one- and two-stage clustered random sampling from a common sampling frame (sampled units are blue wedges)

clusters will be sampled is not known in advance. Indeed, if the survey were to be repeated, different clusters would be sampled. In other words, there is randomness in the clusters selected, while in stratified sampling, there is no randomness in the strata selected. Consequently, in clustered sampling designs, variability comes from both sampling the clusters and sampling within the clusters. These two sources of variability are referred to as *between-cluster* and *within-cluster* variances.

Survey estimates based on a clustered design tend to have higher standard errors than those from a simple random sample with the same sample size. We can already anticipate that clustering will affect total variance because of the need to account for both between- and within-cluster variance. Sometimes the explanation advanced for why clustering inflates variance is that observations within a cluster tend to be similar, so one is not getting as much information from a clustered sample as from a sample in which all elements are independent. To try and gain some insight into this explanation, let's consider an extreme example.

Suppose we are surveying a population to learn about a binary outcome—whether individuals received a flu shot last year—and suppose our clusters are families. For ease of illustration, assume that all families have four members. Suppose also that p =50% of the population received a flu shot but, since families tend to behave similarly, either all members or no members of each family received the shot. Now, suppose we take a survey sample of $n = 100$ individuals. If the population is large and we take a simple random sample, then it is unlikely that we will sample multiple members of the same family, and the variance of our estimate can be calculated based on the binomial distribution as $p(1-p)/\sqrt{n} = 0.25/10 = 0.025$. But if we follow a single-stage clustered design and sample 25 families, the variance of our estimate will be $p(1-p)/\sqrt{25} = 0.25/5 = 0.05$. This calculation reflects that all members of the same cluster have the same outcome, so instead of 100 independent observations, we effectively have only 25. There is no within-cluster variance, so the between-cluster variance 0.05 is the total variance.

Now, consider a two-stage clustered design that samples, for example, two individuals from each of 50 families. This would yield an intermediate variance estimate of $0.25/\sqrt{50} = 0.035$. In general, a two-stage clustered design yields standard errors that depend on both between- and within-cluster variation, but in this example, there is no within-cluster variation since all individuals within a family have the same outcome.

This extreme example illustrates the loss of information that occurs due to similarity of outcomes within clusters and how this loss translates into an inflated variance relative to simple random sampling. In practice, we would expect more variation within families. In some families, only parents might receive a flu shot, in others only children. Still, in a single-stage cluster design, variance estimation will still be based only on between-cluster variation.

To understand variance estimation in cluster designs, recall that the definition of variability in a survey is the fluctuation in estimates if we could repeat the survey many times. In single-stage clustering, we draw different clusters each time, but the per-cluster outcome is fully determined; if the same clusters were to be drawn again, the same outcome would be obtained. In two-stage clustering which samples some, but not all, observations within each cluster, the per-cluster outcome has some randomness to it and could differ on repeated sampling. In this case, standard errors will be a composite of between- and within-cluster variance. The precise formula is less important than the understanding of the sources of variation and how they contribute to increasing variability under a clustered design.

9.7 Variance Estimation and Weighting in Complex Surveys

The designs of large national surveys, such as the NHIS, NHANES, and MEPS, include stratification and multiple levels of clustering. The NHIS stratifies by state and samples geographic regions—metropolitan statistical areas, counties, or groups of contiguous counties—within each state. The geographic clustering is necessary because of the personal interview nature of the survey. Within each geographic region, households are sampled. Thus, the survey followed a stratified, two-stage clustering design. In this design, first-stage clusters (here, geographic regions) are the primary sampling units (PSUs). The second-stage clusters (here, households) which are sampled within each cluster are the *secondary sampling units* (SSUs). The NHIS in 2006–2015 sampled more than 400 PSUs from roughly 1900 units

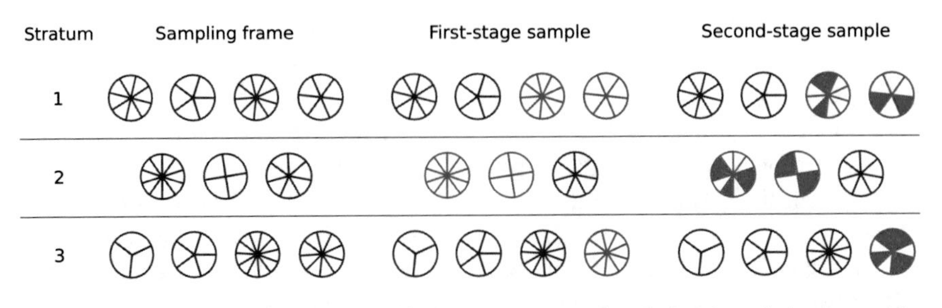

Fig. 9.2 Schematic illustration of a stratified, two-stage sampling design (sampled units are blue wedges)

covering all 50 states and the District of Columbia. The survey was redesigned in 2016 but still follows roughly the same stratified, two-stage scheme [5].

Variance estimation in complex, multistage designs follows from the ideas presented earlier in the sections on stratification and clustering. In a stratified, two-stage design, variances are estimated within strata and summed across strata. Within each stratum, at least two PSUs are needed to properly estimate between-cluster variation. Various ad hoc remedies can be employed when this is not the case. One option is to assume that between-cluster variance is similar in strata with only one PSU and strata with at least two PSUs. Another is to center the data for single-PSU strata at the grand mean for the entire sample.

In multistage designs, design-based weights (called *base weights*) are given by the inverse of the probability of being sampled. Consider the example in Fig. 9.2, which shows a stratified, two-stage sampling design with three strata. To be concrete, let's say that the strata represent three categories of the Census Bureau's urban–rural classification: (1) urbanized areas, (2) urban clusters, and (3) rural [9]. The PSUs are schools (circles) and the SSUs (wedges) are students within schools. Within each stratum, there are three or four potential schools to sample, but the sampling probabilities are not the same within each stratum. The probability of each school being selected is $1/2$ in the first stratum, $2/3$ in the second stratum, and $1/4$ in the third stratum. Thus, the survey oversamples PSUs in the second stratum. Within each school, there is also a stratum-specific probability of sampling students. The probability of each student being selected in a sampled school is $1/3$ in the first stratum, $1/2$ in the second stratum, and $2/3$ in the third stratum. Thus, the probability of being sampled is $1/2 \times 1/3 = 1/6$, $2/3 \times 1/2 = 1/3$, and $1/4 \times 2/3 = 1/6$ in the three strata, and the corresponding base weights for students in these strata are 6, 3, and 6.

Base weights are typically modified by post-stratification, leading to random weights that are ultimately data-dependent. This makes estimating the variance of population-representative summaries a complex problem—we need to account for not only the sample design elements (stratification, clustering) but also the variance of the weights themselves. In the next section, we will try to produce an estimate of the average annual medical expenditure associated with a prior diabetes diagnosis in the United States. If, for each person in a sample, we could observe how much their diabetes costs amounted to in a given year, the formula for the estimate could be written as a weighted average:

$$\text{Estimated average expenditure} = \frac{\sum_{i=1}^{n_i} \widehat{W}_i \widehat{Y}_i}{\sum_{i=1}^{n_i} \widehat{W}_i},$$

where W_i is the sample weight associated with observation i and Y_i is cost of diabetes care for person i. In the next section, we will estimate the average via a regression model, but the key here is to note that the estimated weights enter into both the numerator and denominator of the weighted mean. The denominator, which is the sum of the weights, is an estimate of the number of persons with diabetes in the population. Because the final estimate is a non-linear function of weights and survey data, there is no easy way to calculate the variance.

There are two main approaches for variance estimation based on complex surveys. The first, *linearization*, is based on a mathematical technique, called the *delta method*. This approach uses a Taylor series expansion to approximate the estimate by a linear function of its components. This approximation is justified in large samples. The second approach is based on computational ideas and includes several techniques, all of which create multiple replicates of the original sample data [10]. Computational techniques for variance estimation from complex surveys include balanced repeated replication, the jackknife, and the bootstrap. All of these techniques create replicates of the data. Balanced repeated replication and the jackknife work by omitting some PSUs and reweighting the rest. Then, the original estimation procedure is applied, and the variance is estimated empirically across the replicated datasets. Linearization- and replication-based variance estimation procedures are options in software packages that offer routines for analysis of complex survey samples. In the next section, we demonstrate such an analysis with the goal of estimating the US average and total annual medical expenditures associated with a prior diabetes diagnosis in the United States.

9.8 Analyzing Survey Data: The Cost of Diabetes in the United States

The nation's medical bill due to specific illnesses or conditions is of great interest to many government agencies and policymakers. For example, what are the total costs attributable to diabetes in 2020? How have the costs of care for melanoma changed as expensive new immunotherapies have disseminated in the population? How much of health care spending is attributable to being overweight or obese, and how has this changed over time?

When the condition of interest is clinical and identifiable in medical claims or hospital discharge records, these sources may be used to determine the average costs of care per individual, which can then be scaled up to reflect population expenditures. However, when the condition is subjective or not routinely recorded in administrative data, self-reported information on conditions and medical expenditures can be extremely valuable. Gaskin and Richard [11] used the MEPS 2008 data to study the total medical care costs associated with self-reported chronic pain, including arthritis or joint pain. Biemer et al. [12] used MEPS data from 2006–2013 to study the rising costs of obesity to the US health care system. And Kirkland et al. [13] used MEPS data from 2003 to 2014 to analyze trends in health care expenditures among US adults with hypertension.

In this section, we use MEPS 2017 data to study the annual and total medical expenditures attributable to a (self-reported) prior diagnosis of diabetes. In Chap. 6, we used regression analysis for this purpose, focusing on the specifics of different approaches to handle the extremely non-normal features of the distribution of health cost outcomes. We used MEPS 2017 data but did not address the survey aspects of the sample and instead treated the data if it were a simple random sample. Not anymore!

Our analysis has three objectives: (1) to estimate the number of persons in the United States in 2017 previously diagnosed with diabetes; (2) to estimate average incremental health care costs per person with a prior diagnosis of diabetes compared to those without a prior diagnosis adjusted for age, sex, and race/ethnicity; and (3) to estimate the total incremental costs to the US health care system associated with prevalent diabetes.

As a complex, multistage survey, the public-use MEPS data include variables that provide individual survey weights and survey design variables that can be used in the analysis. Specialized survey analysis software must also be used.

An analysis of survey data begins by specifying the person weights and survey design variables. In the MEPS 2017 data, these are the weight variable (PERWT17F) and the variables specifying strata (VARSTR) and clusters (VARPSU). Once these have been specified, we can address our three objectives.

We first focus on adults (age 18 years or older) and estimate the number with a prior diabetes diagnosis. In the MEPS 2017 data, there are 23,529 adults, of whom 2806 (11.9%) are recorded as having reported a prior diabetes diagnosis. When we scale the sample up to the population using the sample weights, we estimate that 25.7 million individuals have diabetes, amounting to 10.5% of the adult population.

When an analysis of survey data examines a subset of the dataset (e.g., individuals age 18 or older), we do not simply exclude individuals who are not in the subset because doing so would leave a weighted sample that is not representative of the population [14]. Rather, the weights for the remaining subset must be properly adjusted, and this adjustment is done automatically within survey software when given the appropriate commands indicating that the analysis focuses on a subset of the data. In the MEPS analysis, our subset consisted of all inscope individuals age 18 years or older.

Turning now to the question of incremental medical costs, we first estimate the mean incremental cost as the coefficient of the diabetes indicator in a linear regression adjusted for age, sex, and race/ethnicity. The results are shown in Table 9.2.

Table 9.2 Estimated incremental medical costs for persons age 18 years or older in the United States using a naive linear regression and unweighted and weighted regressions that account for the MEPS 2017 survey design, each adjusted for age, sex, and race/ethnicity

Model	Coefficient	95% CI	*P*-value
Naive	7059.16	(6392.19, 7726.14)	<0.001
Unweighted	7059.16	(6075.40, 8042.93)	<0.001
Weighted	6880.92	(5812.08, 7949.76)	<0.001

For comparison, the table shows results using naive linear regression (i.e., unweighted and not accounting for the sampling design) and using either unweighted or weighted regression that accounts for the sampling design. As this example shows, the estimated coefficient of a prior diabetes diagnosis does not depend on the sampling design, but it does depend on the sample weights. Also, the standard error and associated 95% confidence interval depends on both the sampling design and the sample weights.

Next, we multiply the estimated mean incremental cost from the fitted regression by the number of individuals with diabetes in the population. The results imply total annual medical expenditures associated with a prior diabetes diagnosis in the United States in 2017 were $182 billion (unweighted) or $177 billion (weighted). Either estimate is a staggering amount.

It may seem that a weighted regression should be most appropriate, but this is in fact subject to controversy. Korn and Graubard [7] contrast coefficients from weighted and unweighted regressions in an analysis of data from the National Maternal and Infant Health Survey. Their examples show that in the case where the true association between a covariate and an outcome is non-linear, a weighted regression may emphasize a different subrange of the covariates than an unweighted regression, and this will alter the coefficient estimates. But the question of whether to use weighted or unweighted estimates goes far deeper to encompass considerations of efficiency [15], internal consistency, and robustness [16]. In Table 9.2, both weighted and unweighted estimates are presented and produce fairly similar results about the adjusted incremental expenditures among adults with diabetes in the United States.

Standard linear regression provides unbiased estimates of the incremental medical costs associated with a prior diabetes diagnosis. But this model does not account for the highly non-normal distribution of health cost outcomes. When we discussed specialized regression models for health cost outcomes in Chap. 6, we noted that standard linear regression might not generate correct standard errors and confidence intervals. As an alternative, we offered two-part models [17] and marginal effect estimates, with standard errors estimated via bootstrapping. Considerations when estimating predictive margins using survey data are discussed by Graubard and Korn [18]. Marginal effects for two-part models using survey data are provided in Stata's `twopm` package [19], but estimating the variance of these effects is complex. Methods for variance estimation based on survey samples continue to evolve and remain an active area of statistical methodology research.

9.9 Software and Data

R code to download data and to carry out the examples in this book is available at the GitHub page https://roman-gulati.github.io/statistics-for-health-data-science/. In addition to the R packages cited in Chap. 1, this chapter also used the `survey` package [20, 21].

References

1. Centers for Disease Control and Prevention: Diabetes Report Card (a). https://www.cdc.gov/diabetes/library/reports/reportcard/incidence-2017.html. Accessed 11 July 2020
2. Centers for Disease Control and Prevention: National Health Interview Survey (b). http://www.cdc.gov/nchs/nhis/index.htm. Accessed 12 February 2020
3. Centers for Disease Control and Prevention: National Health and Nutrition Examination Survey (c). https://www.cdc.gov/nchs/nhanes/index.htm. Accessed 12 February 2020
4. Agency for Healthcare Research and Quality: Medical Expenditure Panel Survey. http://www.ahrq.gov/research/data/meps/index.html. Accessed 12 February 2020
5. Blewett, L.A., Dahlen, H.A., Spencer, D., Rivera Drew, J.A., Lukanen, E.: Changes to the design of the National Health Interview Survey to support enhanced monitoring of health reform impacts at the state level. Am. J. Public Health **106**, 1961–1966 (2016)
6. United States Census Bureau: American Community Survey (a). https://www.census.gov/programs-surveys/acs. Accessed 11 July 2020
7. Korn, E.L., Graubard, B.I.: Examples of differing weighted and unweighted estimates from a sample survey. Am. Stat. **49**, 291–295 (1995)
8. Lohr, S.: Sampling: Design and Analysis, 2nd edn. Chapman & Hall/CRC Press, New York (2010). https://www.sharonlohr.com/sampling-design-and-analysis
9. United States Census Bureau: Urban and Rural Classifications (b). https://www.census.gov/programs-surveys/geography/guidance/geo-areas/urban-rural/2010-urban-rural.html. Accessed 11 July 2020
10. Kolenikov, S.: Resampling variance estimation for complex survey data. STATA J. **10**(2), 165–199 (2010)
11. Gaskin, D.J., Richard, P.: The economic costs of pain in the United States. J. Pain **13**, 715–724 (2012)
12. Biemer, A., Cawley, J., Meyerhofer, C.: The high and rising costs of obesity to the US health care system. J. Gen. Intern. Med. **32**, 6–8 (2017)
13. Kirkland, E.B., Heincelman, N., Bishu, K.G., Schumann, S.O., Schreiner, A., Axon, R.N., Mauldin, P.D., Moran, W.P.: Trends in healthcare expenditures among US adults with hypertension: National estimates, 2003–2014. J. Am. Heart Assoc. **11**, e008731 (2018)
14. Graubard, B.I., Korn, E.L.: Survey inference for subpopulations. Am. J. Epidemiol. **144**(1), 102–106 (1996)
15. Winship, C., Radbill, L.: Sampling weights and regression analysis. Sociol. Methods Res. **23**, 230–257 (1994)
16. Lohr, S.L.: Comment: Struggles with survey weighting and regression modeling. Stat. Sci. **22**(2), 175–178 (2007)
17. Deb, P., Norton, E.C., Manning, W.G.: Health Econometrics Using Stata. Stata Press, College Station, (2017)
18. Graubard, B.I., Korn, E.L.: Predictive margins with survey data. Biometrics **55**(2), 652–659 (1999)

19. Belotti, F., Deb, P., Manning, W.G., Norton, E.C.: twopm: Two-part models. STATA J. **15**(1), 3–20 (2015)
20. Lumley, T.: Survey analysis in R (). https://r-survey.r-forge.r-project.org/survey/r
21. Lumley, T.: Complex Surveys: A Guide to Analysis Using R. Wiley, New York (2010). https://r-survey.r-forge.r-project.org/svybook/

Chapter 10
Prediction

Abstract This chapter discusses methods for studies in which prediction of health outcomes is a primary goal. Studies that seek to predict are fundamentally different from those that seek to explain. While the analytic methods may overlap, there are many flexible, automated methods that are only appropriate in the prediction setting. We introduce two such approaches, regularized regression and tree-based algorithms, and apply them to predict annual health care costs and hospitalization using Medical Expenditure Panel Survey (MEPS) data given participant characteristics and prior patterns of health care utilization and costs. We emphasize that prediction is about finding a balance between too much and too little flexibility and explain the technique of cross-validation to determine this balance. Ultimately a predictive model is evaluated based on its accuracy in an independent (test) dataset. We review metrics for predictive model performance and use them to evaluate the models for health outcomes in the MEPS dataset.

10.1 Explaining Versus Predicting

In this era of big data, our digital lives generate massive amounts of information that is being harnessed constantly to identify and forecast our needs, wants, and next moves. In health care, longitudinal health surveys catalog health-related behaviors and preferences; medical claims and records capture diagnosis and procedure trajectories; and germline genomic studies generate high-dimensional DNA fingerprints that may help to personalize our medical care. Who will get breast cancer? Who is at high risk of recurrence once diagnosed? Which patients are most likely to decompensate while in intensive care and should therefore be monitored most closely? All these questions are about prediction. In this chapter we study methods for health data analysis where the central goal is prediction.

In 2012, the Heritage Provider Network ran one of the earliest public data science competitions—to predict the number of days individuals would spend in a hospital in the coming year given data from prior years. The text of the competition announcement read:

R. Etzioni et al., *Statistics for Health Data Science*, Springer Texts in Statistics,
https://doi.org/10.1007/978-3-030-59889-1_10

> The winning team will create an algorithm that predicts how many days a patient will spend in a hospital in the next year. Once known, health care providers can develop new care plans and strategies to reach patients before emergencies occur, thereby reducing the number of unnecessary hospitalizations. This will result in increasing the health of patients while decreasing the cost of care. In short, a winning solution will change health care delivery as we know it—from an emphasis on caring for the individual after they get sick to a true health care system.

Later in this chapter we will return to these aspirations and discuss whether they can be achieved using predictive algorithms. Since the Heritage Health Prize, such crowdsourcing competitions have become commonplace. Teams compete to predict a specified outcome and are ranked according to the accuracy of their algorithm on external data not used to develop it.

In previous chapters, we studied methods for inference, with our primary objective being to understand the data-generating mechanism. For an outcome like hospitalization, we would harness regression modeling to identify the factors that explain why certain people are more likely to be hospitalized than others. The factors explored would likely have been cast within a conceptual model that acknowledged confounders or mediators. We would select a statistical model that is appropriate for the outcome, formulate well-defined hypotheses, and implement the corresponding inferential procedures.

What if our goal is not to explain but to predict? In other words, we are not focused on explaining the data or testing hypotheses; we just want to predict the outcome, here hospitalization, as accurately as possible. We may have a large set of patient factors and other variables in our data; which specific variables explain the variation in patient outcomes does not matter as much as how well they combine to identify high- and low-risk patients. We may, and often will, resort to an automated algorithm to figure out which combination works best. When we are done, the combination itself matters less than how well it predicts; predictive accuracy is key. We have transitioned from models to algorithms.

A familiar automated algorithm that uses the machinery of the preceding chapters is stepwise regression. Stepwise regression is a procedure for variable selection in a setting where there is a large set of predictor variables and no specific conceptual model for how to determine which ones are to be included or excluded. In *forward stepwise* regression, variables are considered one at a time, and a variable is added if its p-value is below a specified threshold given the variables already in the model. Once all the outstanding variables stop satisfying this criterion, the model is considered complete. A *backward stepwise* algorithm takes out variables one at a time using similar but reverse logic: eliminate a variable when its p-value is above a specified threshold. While stepwise regression generates a bona fide regression model, the multiple testing and the customization of the selected set of variables to the sample data make the procedure completely invalid for inference; it cannot be used to explain. The problem is articulately summarized as follows [1]: "your parameter estimates are likely to be too far away from zero, your variance estimates for those parameter estimators are not correct either, so confidence intervals and hypothesis tests will be wrong, and there are no reasonable ways of correcting these problems."

The dichotomy between explaining and predicting is perfectly captured by Leo Breiman's seminal paper [2] published in 2001 on the two cultures of statistical analysis: models and algorithms. The models culture corresponds to the goal of explaining. In this culture, the notion is that the data are generated by a specific model that must be accommodated by the analytic procedure. Medical expenditures data with a spike at zero should preferably be analyzed using a two-part model rather than a least squares model. Overdispersed count outcomes should preferably be analyzed via negative binomial rather than Poisson regression. We must respect the data-generating model so we can trust our inferences that are in service to the goal of explaining it. In the algorithms culture, we do not know or necessarily care what model generated the data; we just want to predict well. In 2001, the statistical world was essentially entrenched in the first culture. Breiman's paper was about the need to integrate the second culture into their practice because, by confining themselves to the first culture, they were in danger of missing important opportunities to make their science relevant to the big data era.

In the algorithms culture, how predictors affect the outcome is essentially a black box; see Fig. 10.1. While the models culture would try to understand the black box, making it as transparent as possible, the algorithms culture ignores the box and is all about the leap from the predictors to the outcome. Of course, the modeling approach can use the estimated model to predict the outcome, but it is typically limited to relatively simple models. By giving up the need to explicitly formulate the mechanism inside the black box and create a model that is valid for inference, the algorithmic approach can harness complex algorithms that may not even be possible to formulate mathematically.

While predictive algorithms can be more flexible and potentially more accurate, an algorithm that predicts the data at hand too closely may be useless for predicting new data. This is the problem of overfitting. Before presenting some common prediction techniques, we first describe the problem of overfitting and introduce accuracy metrics that are typically used to evaluate the performance of predictive algorithms. While we generally use the term "algorithms" to refer to analytic techniques when prediction is the goal, we sometimes use the terms "predictive models" and "predictive algorithms" interchangeably.

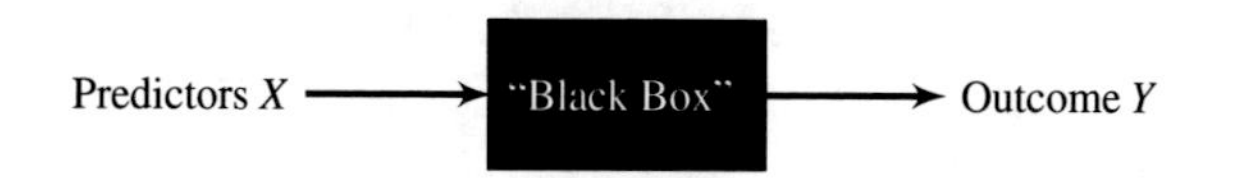

Fig. 10.1 Data generating mechanism—do we really need to understand the black box?

10.2 Overfitting and the Bias-Variance Tradeoff

When the goal is to predict, we can fit any analytic model to a dataset without being concerned about its interpretability or complexity. This means that, with a sufficiently rich set of predictors and an adequately complex model, we can achieve a perfect fit—an algorithm that exactly and successfully "predicts" the outcome for any individual in the data. However, this perfect performance on the observed dataset may not, and most likely never will, be realized when applying the model to new data, which is the main purpose, and indeed the very definition, of prediction.

To demonstrate overfitting, we revisit the problem of age as a predictor of body mass index (BMI) discussed in Chap. 3. The data are from the National Health and Nutrition Examination Survey (NHANES) [3], which comprises a representative sample from the US population and includes self-reported information as well as empirical health status measures, such as body mass index (BMI) and blood pressure. NHANES has been an authoritative source for trends in health characteristics in the United States, including obesity, diabetes, and hypertension, for the last several decades.

We use data on 1000 individuals age 2–80 years from the NHANES 2015 sample and fit a series of models with a single predictor (age) but with increasing complexity. We consider only models where age is grouped into equal-length intervals, ranging from 2 intervals of lengths 39 and 40 years to 79 intervals of length 1 year each. Figure 10.2 shows predictions of the models with 2 and 79 groups over a scatterplot of age and BMI. The 2-group model (green) is inflexible, so it does not capture the general relationship across ages, particularly in children and older persons. The 79-group model (blue) is more flexible; its global shape captures the general relationship across the range of ages better, but its local behavior is quite noisy.

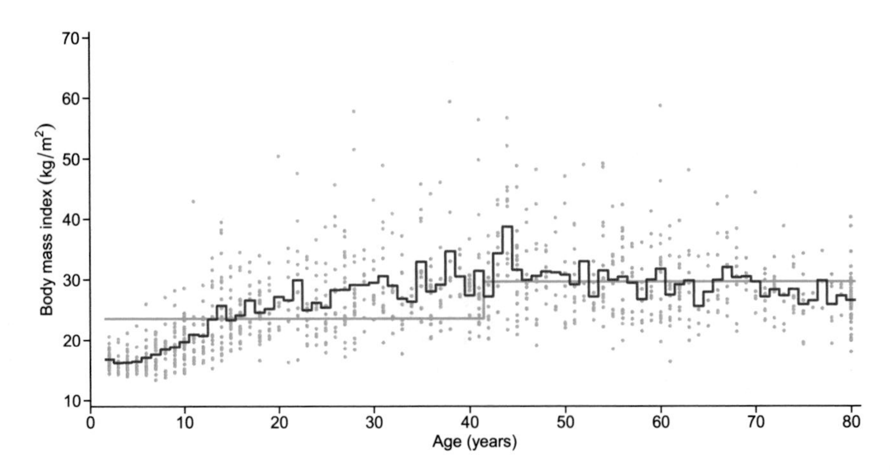

Fig. 10.2 Fitted linear regressions for body mass index given age split into 2 (green) or 79 (blue) groups based on 1000 observations from the NHANES 2015 data

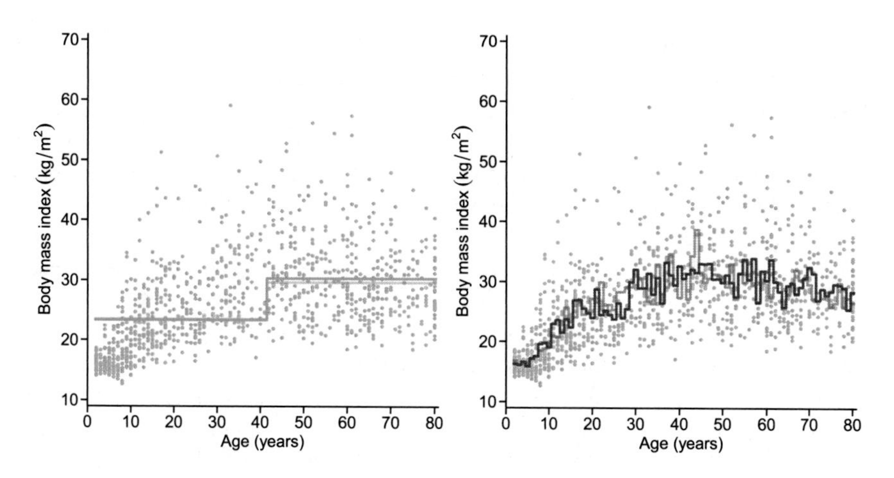

Fig. 10.3 Fitted linear regressions for body mass index given age split into 2 (green) or 79 (blue) subgroups based on 1000 observations (opaque) with predicted values from the models fit to the previous sample of 1000 observations (semi-transparent) from the NHANES 2015 data

Figure 10.3 shows the same models fit to an independent set of 1000 individuals from the NHANES 2015 data. The predictions from Fig. 10.2 for the original set appear in the plots as semi-transparent lines. While the 2-group predictions are very similar, the 79-group predictions are very different for many ages. The 79-group predictions show the same global pattern that increases, stabilizes, and then starts to decrease with age, but they spike at different ages due to random fluctuations between samples.

This is an example of a general phenomenon: models that are too flexible are likely to be influenced by specific observations in a dataset. This phenomenon is known as *overfitting*. When there is overfitting, the model is tailored to the random variation of the data above and beyond any underlying structure. More flexible models capture the randomness in the dataset and may end up predicting less accurately in a new dataset. We refer to the data used for fitting as the *training* data and the new data (used for validation) as the *test* data. The observations shown in Fig. 10.2 may be thought of as training data for the 2- and 79-group models, and those plotted in Fig. 10.3 may be thought of as test data.

The problem of overfitting brings us to a key principle in predictive analytics: the *bias-variance tradeoff*. Bias refers to a model's inability to capture the underlying truth, not because of sampling errors but due to the assumptions made in its construction. Variance refers to the variability in a model's predictions across datasets from a population with a given underlying truth. The bias-variance tradeoff is demonstrated visually in Fig. 10.3. Theoretically, if we fit the same model to many independent datasets drawn from the same population, a prediction from a more flexible model will tend to be closer on average to the truth and hence will have a smaller bias. However, the variance of model's predictions in different data sets will be larger. In this example, the 2-group model has a small variance—it produces similar predictions when applied to independent samples, but it does not capture the underlying truth of the age–BMI relationship well; it has large bias. Conversely, the 79-group model has large variance but small bias.

Bias and variance are a consequence of model flexibility—a model that is too flexible increases variance, while a model that is not flexible enough increases bias. Recognizing this tradeoff is fundamental because it motivates the need to identify a compromise. In practice, we seek a model with the right amount of flexibility that will lead to reliably accurate predictive performance in datasets that were not used to estimate the model.

The bias-variance sweet spot may depend on the size of the dataset used to build the predictive model. Increasing the sample size will have little or no effect on the bias of the 2-group and 79-group models analyzed above, but it can dramatically reduce their variances. With larger sample sizes, increased model flexibility comes at a lower cost in terms of model variance. Thus, for larger datasets, we can use more flexible, complex, and accurate models, and this is a key reason for the popularity of flexible machine learning methods like deep learning in the era of big data.

10.3 Evaluating Predictive Performance

When we study a prediction problem, our goal is invariably to predict outcomes for new observations—either predicting future outcomes or, as in the Heritage Health Prize problem, predicting outcomes in a new dataset not used to develop the algorithm. Generally speaking, the performance of a prediction algorithm on the training data is much less interesting than its performance on the test data. Indeed, based on our discussion of bias and variance, it should not be surprising that we can easily optimize predictive performance on the training data by selecting the most flexible algorithm available.

We begin by defining a common metric to measure performance of a predictive model. The mean squared error (MSE) is the average squared difference between an observed outcome and a prediction:

$$\text{MSE} = \text{Average}(\text{Predicted} - \text{Observed})^2.$$

The closer the prediction is to the outcome, the smaller the MSE and the better the performance of the model. Figure 10.4 shows MSEs of linear regressions for BMI given age split into different numbers of age groups. The figure shows two sets of MSEs—one set is calculated for the training data (semi-transparent), using the same observations that were used to fit the model, and the other set is calculated for the test data (opaque). Because the variance of BMI differs slightly between the two datasets, we standardize the MSEs by dividing them by the variance of BMI.

As expected, the MSEs calculated for the training data decrease with the complexity of the model. In other words, the more flexible the model, the better it performs when predicting the same observations used to build it. This is not

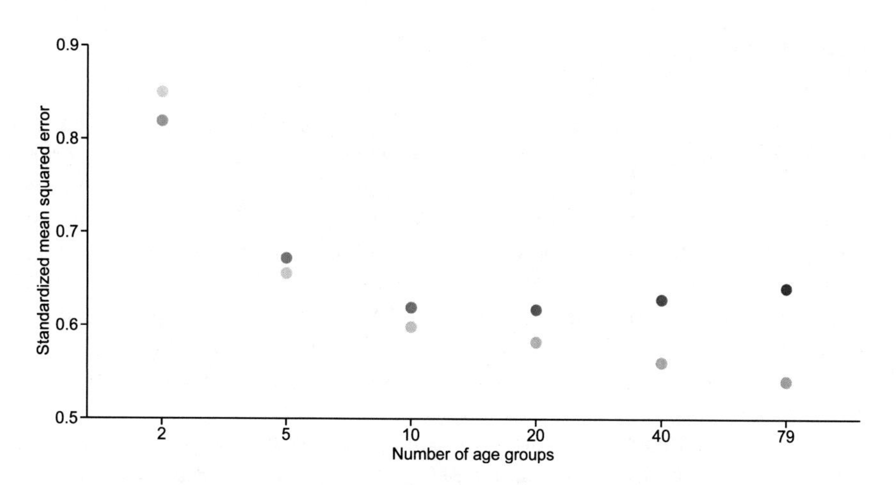

Fig. 10.4 Standardized mean squared errors of linear regression models for body mass index given age split into selected numbers of age groups evaluated using training data (semi-transparent) or test data (opaque)

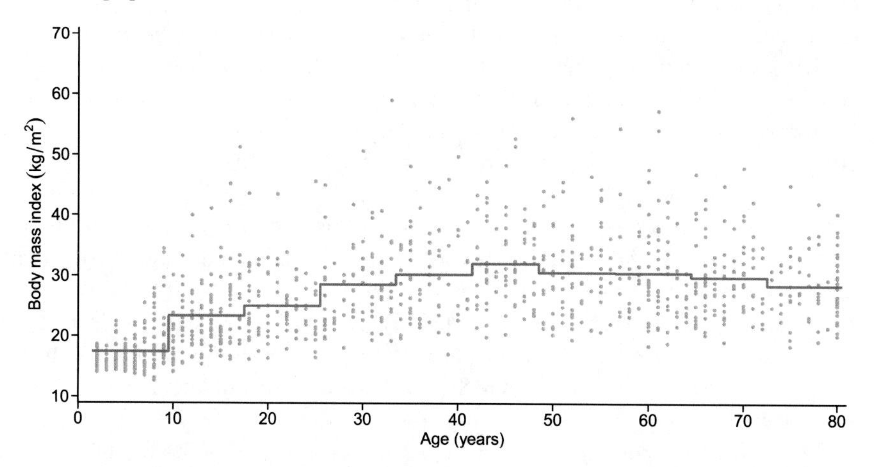

Fig. 10.5 Predictions from the 10-group model fit to training data and applied to test data

surprising as the model is fit via least squares, so its parameters were chosen to minimize the MSE. Also, in all cases except the 2-group model, the performance on the training data is better than on the test data.

In contrast, the predictive performance on the test data initially improves with the complexity of the model, but then it worsens as the number of groups approaches 79. The best performers based on the test data are the models with 10 or 20 age groups rather than the one with the full 79 groups. Figure 10.5 presents the 10-group model fit to the training data and used to predict BMI in the test data. The 10-group model is smoother than the 79-group model presented in Fig. 10.3. It compromises well between bias and variance, giving the best predictive performance for the test data across the models evaluated.

10.4 Cross-Validation

Figure 10.4 shows that performance assessment using independent test data can help determine the level of flexibility to optimize predictive performance. However, we do not always have the luxury of being able to sample two datasets for the purpose of model development; further, partitioning an available training dataset into a portion for training and a portion for testing can lead to considerable loss of information for model fitting. *Cross-validation* is a general technique that uses all training observations for both model fitting and performance assessment, permitting selection of a model that is likely to perform well when predicting on new data and controlling the problem of overfitting. We present the basics of the technique here; more discussion and examples can be found in James et al. [4].

Cross-validation is used to select a specific model from a series of models that differ in their flexibility. In predicting BMI given age, we might have six models, each with a different number of age groups, and we can use cross-validation to identify the optimal number of groups to include. This idea can be generalized to encompass any predictive algorithm that is indexed by a *flexibility parameter* (here the number of age groups), also called a *tuning* or *complexity parameter*.

Cross-validation randomly partitions the data into K sub-datasets, or *folds*, of similar size, fits a given model to the data in the first $K - 1$ folds, and evaluates its performance using the Kth fold, storing the resulting MSE. The training dataset comprises the first $K - 1$ folds and the test dataset comprises the Kth fold. This generalizes what we did in the previous section with the training and test datasets with $K = 2$. In cross-validation, we repeat this process K times, each time removing one of the folds, fitting the model to the remaining data, and calculating the performance measure on the unused fold. This yields K different values of the performance measure, MSE(1), MSE(2), ..., MSE(K). The key is that the performance measure is evaluated using observations that were not used to fit the model. The overall cross-validated MSE is calculated by averaging over the K fold-specific MSE values.

The entire procedure is implemented for each candidate model in our series of models. In the case of the BMI prediction problem, suppose we have six candidate models, each with a different number of age groups. This would produce six cross-validated MSEs, and we would choose the model (i.e., the number of age groups) that yields the smallest of these values. We would then fit this selected model to the entire training dataset. Thus, cross-validation does not give us the final model for predicting outcomes in the test data; rather, it gives us the optimal value of the flexibility parameter to be used when fitting the model to the training data.

What number of folds should be used? One approach is to take K equal to the number of observations, so that each model is fit to all observations save one and evaluated on the single observation that was left out. However, this *leave-one-out cross-validation* can be demanding computationally since the number of fitted models equals the number of observations. Further, while the resulting estimate of predictive performance is nearly unbiased, it turns out that its variance is larger

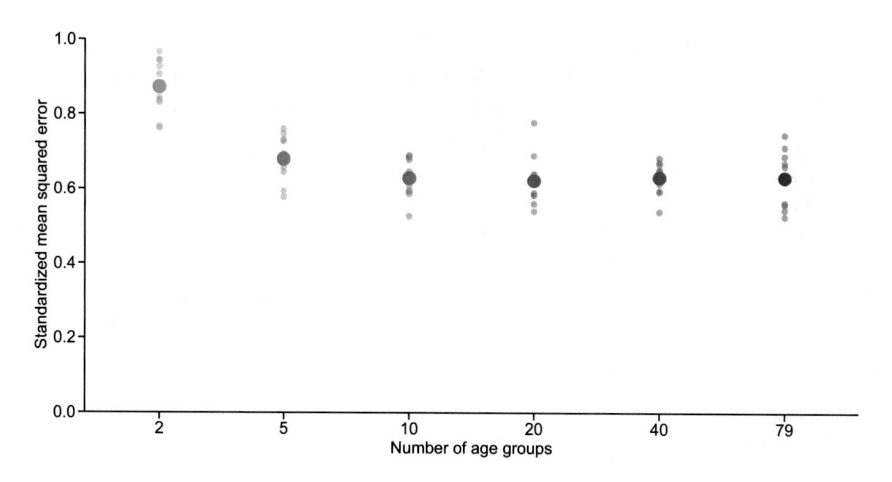

Fig. 10.6 Results of 10-fold cross-validation on six models for body mass index given age split into equal-sized subgroups using 1000 observations from the NHANES 2015 data

than other choices of K [4]. For these reasons, practitioners typically use a smaller number of folds, say $K = 5$ or $K = 10$, depending on the problem and the size of the training dataset.

Figure 10.6 presents the results of 10-fold cross-validation of six candidate models in the BMI example. The data were split into $K = 10$ folds with 100 observations in each, and each of the 6 models was fit 10 times, each time calculating the MSE on the held-out fold. The small circles in the figure show the 10 resulting MSEs, and the large circles show their average, which is the cross-validated MSE, for each model. The performance of the models with 10 and 20 groups is similar, suggesting that either of these could be used for prediction purposes.

This example helps to establish the steps involved in any predictive analysis.

Step 1: Select the outcome variable and the set of predictors, also called *features*, that will potentially be used to predict the outcome.

Step 2: Determine the performance measure that is to be optimized. The specific measure chosen will likely depend on the type of outcome, specifically whether it is binary/categorical or continuous. When the outcome is binary or categorical, the prediction task is generally referred to as *classification*.

Step 3: Identify the set of predictive algorithms and the flexibility parameter. This step amounts to selecting the type of predictive algorithm that will be used.

Step 4: Use cross-validation to identify the value of the flexibility parameter that yields optimal predictive performance.

Step 5: Refit the algorithm using the optimal value of the flexibility parameter to the entire training dataset.

Although the models fit during cross-validation in step 4 can be very different, the final model is the one fit in step 5. The aim of the cross-validation step (step 4) is to choose the flexibility parameter for the final model in step 5. Sometimes, the data are split at the outset into training and test sets, and the algorithm described above uses only the training set. The performance of the model fit in step 5 is then evaluated on the test data as a true measure of predictive performance.

In the following sections, we introduce two types of prediction algorithms. The first, regularized regression, provides an automated version of variable selection in regression models. The second, tree-based algorithms, consists of models that flexibly partition the multidimensional feature space. While these are only two approaches in the vast and growing universe of predictive approaches, they build naturally on the modeling background from earlier chapters and illustrate how predictive analyses are conducted in practice.

10.5 Regularized Regression

When there are many potential predictors, comparing all possible models is tedious and often infeasible. We previously discussed stepwise regression, which is not only inefficient but also examines only a subset of all potential models. Regularized regression is an automated way of selecting a regression model with optimal flexibility, where the model with all predictors is the most flexible and the one with no predictors is the least flexible. There are different versions of regularized regression depending on how we think of the space of models on the flexibility continuum. Regularized regression can be applied to all regression models discussed in previous chapters, but we will focus here on linear regression for continuous outcomes and illustrate the key idea using the age–BMI example.

10.5.1 The Age–BMI Example

The piecewise constant regression models for BMI considered above grouped individuals by the predictor (age) and predicted the outcome (BMI) using the average value of the outcome within each grouping. Computationally, this is done by defining dummy variables to indicate group membership and using these as predictors in the regression. Let's define these variables so that the coefficients (βs) indicate differences between consecutive age groups. In a four-group model, ages could be split into the groups 2–20, 21–40, 41–60, and 61–80; this leads to three dummy variables defined as:

$$\text{Over20} = \begin{cases} 0 & \text{Age} \leq 20 \\ 1 & \text{Age} > 20 \end{cases}$$

$$\text{Over40} = \begin{cases} 0 & \text{Age} \leq 40 \\ 1 & \text{Age} > 40 \end{cases}$$

$$\text{Over60} = \begin{cases} 0 & \text{Age} \le 60 \\ 1 & \text{Age} > 60 \end{cases},$$

and the linear model is formulated as:

$$\text{BMI} = \beta_0 + \beta_1 \times \text{Over20} + \beta_2 \times \text{Over40} + \beta_3 \times \text{Over60} + \epsilon,$$

where, as usual, ϵ is the error term. A person younger than 20 years old has the value 0 for all three variables Over20, Over40, and Over60, and hence his/her predicted BMI is β_0. A person belonging to the next age group 21–40 has Over20 set to 1 and the other two variables set to 0, so his/her predicted BMI is $\beta_0 + \beta_1$. Thus, β_1 is simply the difference between the predicted BMI in the first and second age groups. Similar reasoning leads to recognizing that β_2 and β_3 are differences in the predicted BMI between age groups 21–40 and 41–60 and between 41–60 and 61–80, respectively. Of course, to fit models with more age groups, one should construct more dummy variables, and the βs will correspond to the differences in BMI between consecutive groups.

There is a direct link between the smoothness of a prediction model as formulated above and its β coefficients. In Fig. 10.2, two prediction models are plotted. The blue step function summarizes the predictions from the 79-group model, with each step corresponding to a β coefficient in that model. As previously observed, the model is erratic and has a high variance. This is not surprising as it is the most flexible model. Less flexible models would be expected to be smoother; in a sense, they would fall somewhere in between the 79-group model and a constant model in which all the coefficients (except β_0) are zero. One way to produce such an in-between model would be to force its β coefficients to be smaller in absolute value or, in statistical terms, to *shrink the coefficients toward zero*. This is exactly what regularized regression methods do.

As explained in Chap. 3, linear regression identifies the line closest to the outcome values by minimizing the squared errors. Mathematically, it minimizes the sum:

$$\sum_{i=1}^{n} (\text{Outcome}_i - \text{Predicted}_i)^2 ,$$

where the sum is over all n observations in the data and Predicted_i is the regression line $\beta_0 + \beta_1 X_{1i} + \cdots + \beta_p X_{pi}$ based on the p predictors and their coefficients. To shrink the coefficients toward zero, one can penalize the sum of squared errors by including a term that becomes large when the βs are large and then minimizing the penalized sum of squared errors. The *least absolute shrinkage and selection operator* (LASSO) finds the βs that minimize:

$$\text{LASSO:} \qquad \sum_{i=1}^{n} (\text{Outcome}_i - \text{Predicted}_i)^2 + \lambda \left(|\beta_1| + |\beta_2| + \cdots + |\beta_p| \right).$$

The LASSO tries to compromise between fitting a function close to the observations (by making the first term small) and fitting a function with small steps (by making the second term small). The flexibility parameter λ controls the balance between the two. If $\lambda = 0$, there is no penalty, and the full model (i.e., the model with 79 coefficients in the age–BMI example) is estimated. As λ increases, the penalty term gains importance, and the coefficients are shrunk toward zero. The formulation of the penalty as a function of the absolute values of the regression coefficients leads to some of the coefficients being shrunk all the way to zero. Thus, the LASSO is effectively a predictor selection algorithm. As in stepwise regression, we must be cautious not to over-interpret the specific predictors selected; we discuss this caveat in greater depth later in this section.

A second commonly used regularized regression approach, called *ridge regression*, uses a different penalty. It estimates the βs by minimizing:

$$\text{Ridge:} \qquad \sum_{i=1}^{n} (\text{Outcome}_i - \text{Predicted}_i)^2 + \lambda \left(\beta_1^2 + \beta_2^2 + \cdots + \beta_p^2\right).$$

The form of the penalty leads to the estimated βs being shrunk toward zero, but they do not end up being exactly zero as in the LASSO. The two approaches can be easily applied to various models for continuous, binary, and count data using statistical software packages. However, there is still the question of what value of λ to use. This is where cross-validation comes in handy. Indeed, λ is the flexibility parameter in these models, with large values leading to high bias and small values leading to high variance. Selecting λ is therefore a problem that is tailor-made for cross-validation. We partition the data into K folds, and, for each of a set of λ values, we estimate the corresponding models K times, finally selecting the value of λ that minimizes the cross-validated MSE.

Regularized regression is demonstrated in Fig. 10.7 on the BMI data using as predictors the dummy variables defining all 79 age groups. The semi-transparent step function is the prediction without any regularization shown above in Fig. 10.3. The green and purple lines show predictions for models fit with LASSO and ridge penalties, respectively. The two regularized models agree quite well, but the ridge prediction has many more small steps, while the LASSO prediction has fewer, larger ones.

10.5.2 Regularized Regression with Many Predictors: Hospitalization in MEPS

Regularized regression can be applied to predict outcomes in any regression setting with many predictors. As an example, we consider the problem of predicting hospitalization using data from the Medical Expenditure Panel Survey (MEPS) [5]. The MEPS database was described in Chap. 1. It includes information on

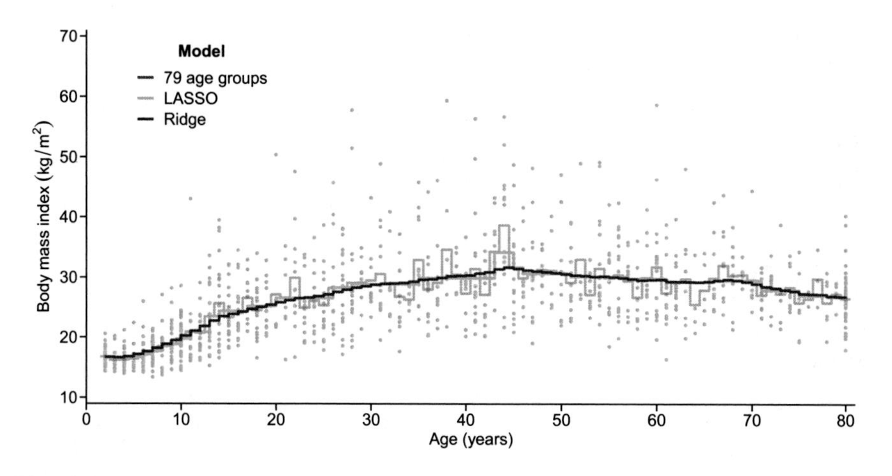

Fig. 10.7 Predictions from linear regressions for body mass index given up to 79 age groups with no penalty (semi-transparent), LASSO penalty (green), or ridge penalty (purple) from 1000 observations from the NHANES 2015 data

participants' socio-demographics, health behaviors, existing conditions, access to care, health care utilization, and expenditures. In this chapter, we use longitudinal MEPS data from a single panel spanning calendar years 2016–2017. Because individuals were followed for 2 years, we can predict outcomes in 2017 using data from the same individuals in 2016.

The MEPS 2016–2017 panel data contains 10,908 individuals who were aged 18 years or older in 2016 after omitting observations with missing values for our predictor variables. We predict hospitalization during 2017 using a logistic regression model given age; sex; race; marital status; family income; education; type of insurance coverage; prior diagnosis with angina, arthritis, asthma, cancer, coronary heart disease, diabetes, emphysema, heart attack, high cholesterol, high blood pressure, heart disease, other heart disease, or stroke; perceived general and mental health status; and any hospitalization in 2016.

Of the 10,908 individuals, 830 (7.6%) were hospitalized during 2017. The results of a standard logistic regression without regularization are compared to logistic regression with LASSO and ridge penalties in Table 10.1. In either regularized regression, the tuning parameter λ for the penalty term was selected by 10-fold cross-validation, and the model results presented are for the entire (training) dataset. For ease of comparison, the coefficients (excluding the intercept) are plotted in Fig. 10.8 from left to right in the same order they appear in the table. The LASSO and ridge regression coefficients are consistently closer to zero than the corresponding coefficients from the standard logistic regression. Also, many of the LASSO coefficients are zero, and non-zero coefficients tend to be closer to the corresponding coefficients from the standard logistic regression than are the coefficients from the ridge regression.

Table 10.1 Fitted standard, LASSO, and ridge regression models to predict hospitalization for persons age 18 years or older in 2017 using longitudinal MEPS 2016–2017 data

Predictor	Standard	LASSO	Ridge
Intercept	−3.901	−3.231	−3.138
Age	0.006	0.003	0.003
Sex = Female	0.399	0.058	0.099
Race = Black	−0.035	0.000	0.017
Race = Amer Indian/Alaska Native	0.352	0.000	0.059
Race = Asian/Native Hawaiian/Pacific Islander	−0.342	0.000	−0.085
Race = Mixed	0.646	0.000	0.190
Married = Widowed	0.270	0.151	0.211
Married = Divorced	−0.039	0.000	0.044
Married = Separated	0.143	0.000	0.077
Married = Never married	−0.119	0.000	−0.053
Poverty = Near poor	−0.486	0.000	−0.049
Poverty = Low income	−0.259	0.000	−0.004
Poverty = Middle income	−0.260	0.000	−0.029
Poverty = High income	−0.257	0.000	−0.045
Education = 9+	0.184	0.000	0.017
Education = 12+	−0.008	0.000	−0.010
Education = 13+	0.098	0.000	−0.009
Education = 16+	−0.089	0.000	−0.034
Insurance = Public only	0.265	0.203	0.137
Insurance = Uninsured	−0.248	0.000	−0.085
Angina diagnosis = Yes	0.716	0.539	0.280
Asthma diagnosis = Yes	0.188	0.000	0.124
Arthritis diagnosis = Yes	0.180	0.237	0.153
Cancer diagnosis = Yes	0.166	0.000	0.141
Coronary heart disease diagnosis = Yes	−0.100	0.000	0.280
Diabetes diagnosis = Yes	0.269	0.182	0.179
Emphysema diagnosis = Yes	0.873	0.709	0.545
Heart attack diagnosis = Yes	0.394	0.295	0.317
High blood pressure diagnosis = Yes	0.357	0.294	0.150
High cholesterol diagnosis = Yes	−0.063	0.000	0.082
Other heart disease diagnosis = Yes	0.412	0.327	0.239
Stroke diagnosis = Yes	0.267	0.130	0.239
Perceived health = Very good	0.129	0.000	−0.059
Perceived health = Good	0.391	0.000	0.017
Perceived health = Fair	0.647	0.217	0.182
Perceived health = Poor	0.718	0.180	0.278
Mental health = Very good	−0.088	0.000	−0.023
Mental health = Good	−0.165	0.000	0.015
Mental health = Fair	0.123	0.056	0.172
Mental health = Poor	−0.165	0.000	0.131
Hospitalized in 2016 = Yes	0.870	0.795	0.419

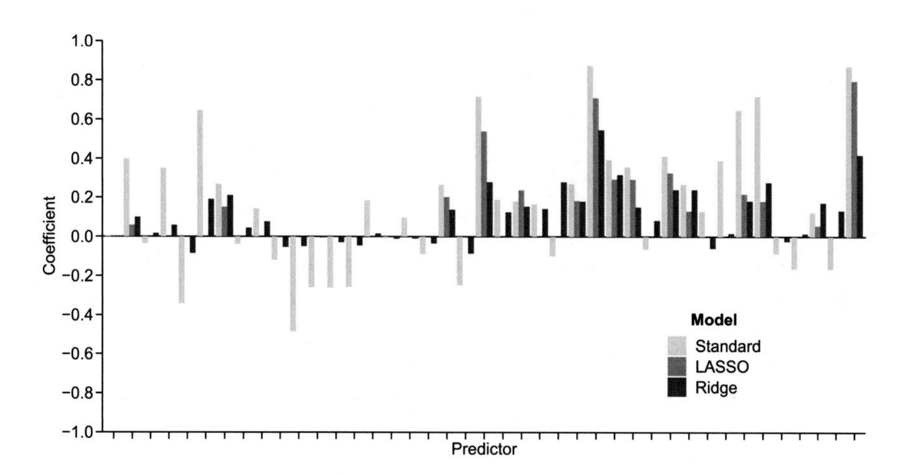

Fig. 10.8 Barplot of the coefficients from the logistic regressions in Table 10.1

In regularized regression models, it is important to define dummy variables in a suitable way. Specifically, if a continuous variable such as age or years of education is split into groups, the variables should be defined as described in Sect. 10.5.1 and not in the more standard way based on indicators of subgroup membership.

Since regularized regression produces a regression model, it may be tempting to use the results to draw inference about associations between predictors and the outcome. This should be done with care for several reasons. First, the coefficient estimates have been shrunk toward zero. They are therefore biased and should not be interpreted as reflecting the true extent of association with the outcome. Second, as in the case of stepwise regression, standard errors and confidence intervals based on the fitted model are not to be trusted. A legitimate use of LASSO results would be to enter the selected predictors in a new regression model fit to an independent test dataset. Ultimately, regularized regression is a predictive algorithm, so the fitted model is not readily useful or valid for inferential purposes.

10.6 Tree-Based Methods

Regression, whether regularized or not, provides a familiar model formulation that we have harnessed in this chapter for prediction purposes. But many predictive algorithms do not lend themselves to closed-form mathematical formulations. In this section, we introduce tree-based methods [6] for prediction or classification; these methods do not produce prediction functions that can be readily written down. The simplest versions do however lend themselves to graphical representations that reflect the essential concept, namely, to identify subsets of the data—based on combinations of their predictor values—with similar values of the outcome and to define the prediction function over these subsets. We return to the age–BMI example from the NHANES data to illustrate the idea.

10.6.1 The Age–BMI Example

In Sect. 10.2, we split age into groups of equal-length intervals and fit step functions using standard regression. Using this approach, the predicted outcome is simply the average BMI in each age group. It is worth noting that we made a choice when we used equal-length intervals (e.g., the 2-group model involved splitting ages into 2–41 and 42–80), and other ways of partitioning age into two groups are possible.

What if another partitioning is preferable? We did not previously explore this. It turns out that, in the case of two groups, using intervals for ages 2–12 and 13–80 yields the largest reduction in MSE (about 33.8%) relative to a 1-group (i.e., intercept-only) model. Thus, this partitioning of the age range is preferable to the partition that bisects the range.

Tree-based methods are all about optimal partitioning. In fact, these algorithms partition recursively, so once the best split of the data into two groups is achieved, each of those groups is again optimally partitioned, where optimal here means "achieving the greatest improvement in accuracy relative to the prior partition." If accuracy is measured via the MSE, then the optimal partition would be the one that results in the largest reduction in MSE.

In the age–BMI example, following the first optimal partitioning of age into two groups, we can look for the next partition that splits either of the groups further and results in the largest reduction in MSE. This again is a simple search that yields the age groups 2–12, 13–25, and 26–80. Prediction using this 3-group model has an MSE that is smaller by about 6.7% than that of the 2-group model. We can continue in the same spirit and find the best 4-group model to be 2–12, 13–25, 26–70, and 71–80 with a further reduction of 1.8% in MSE.

This recursive process of partitioning can continue, yielding a smaller MSE after each iteration. However, it makes sense to stop the process when the reduction in MSE becomes small enough that it does not justify another partition. It might already be clear that not stopping could result in spurious partitions that will ultimately amount to overfitting; we return to this point shortly.

The process of splitting the data into subsets via recursive partitioning can be graphically represented as a tree, with annotation defining the splitting criterion at each point. Each terminal node of the tree represents the subset of the data defined by the series of splits leading to that node. To predict an outcome for an individual, the tree is scanned to locate the terminal subset matching that individual's covariates, and their prediction is given by the average outcome in that subset. Thus, tree-based prediction amounts to a step function over the predictor space, where the locations of the steps are defined by the recursive splits and the values of the step function are given by averages over the corresponding subsets of the data.

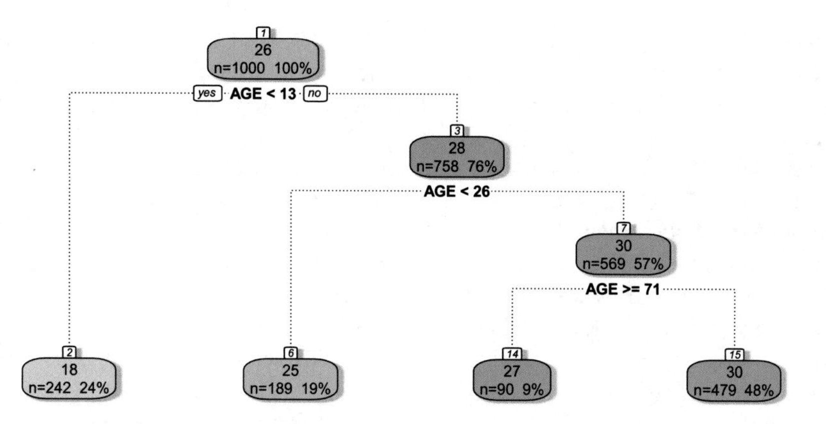

Fig. 10.9 Regression tree for body mass index based on 1000 observations from the NHANES 2015 data

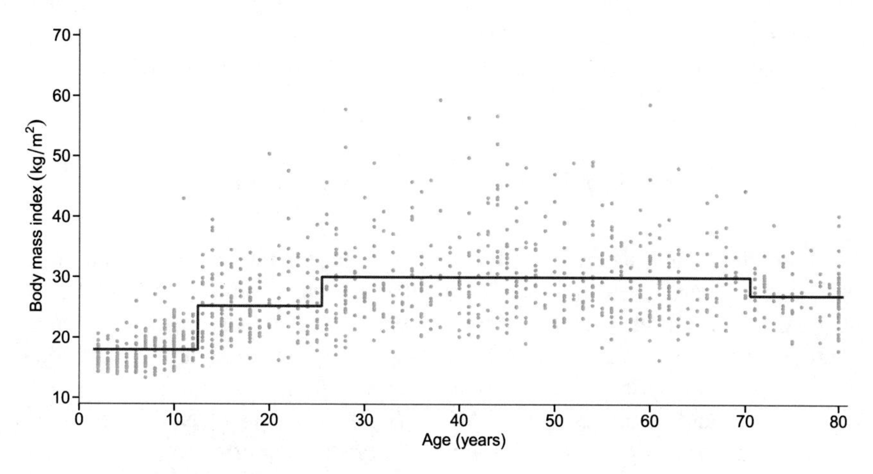

Fig. 10.10 Predictions from the regression tree for body mass index shown in Fig. 10.9

In our age–BMI example, stopping after three splits produces the tree in Fig. 10.9. The tree exactly recapitulates the partitioning process. Starting from the top, at node number 1, we have $n = 1000$ patients whose average BMI is 26. The first partition step splits the data into ages younger versus older than 13 years. At each node, we estimate the average BMI and note the corresponding number and percentage of individuals. This continues until the process ends with four terminal nodes. These are the final groups that the algorithm produces, and the predictions are given by the average outcome in each group. Figure 10.10 superimposes predictions from the four-node tree on the scatterplot of age and BMI.

In general, a larger tree, which has more splits and more terminal nodes, corresponds to a more flexible algorithm, and a smaller tree to a less flexible algorithm. Thus, the flexibility of the algorithm is linked with the size of the tree. Growing larger trees will result in a better performance on training data, but this comes at the risk of poorer generalization to independent data. To reduce the risk of overfitting, the tree can be grown and then pruned, penalizing the complexity of larger trees in a manner similar to the regularized regression models presented earlier.

In practice, there are two tuning parameters that control the size of the tree. The first is a threshold T on the improvement in MSE when growing a tree. If the change in the MSE is less than T, then no more splits are made. A larger value for T is conservative and implies that only splits leading to a substantive change in accuracy are to be considered. While this yields smaller trees and avoids overfitting, it may be short-sighted: a seemingly worthless split early on in the tree might be followed by a very good one later on. Consequently, T is generally set to a low value, and a larger tree is grown first, but then it is judiciously pruned. The second tuning parameter, α, controls the pruning. This parameter takes the form of a penalty on the size of the tree; the tree is pruned to minimize MSE $+ \alpha|N|$, where N is the number of terminal nodes in the tree. A larger value of α incurs a larger penalty for complexity and leads to a smaller pruned tree than a smaller value of α. Next, we examine how this process plays out in the setting of multiple predictors using the MEPS data.

10.6.2 A Regression Tree with Many Predictors

In the setting of multiple predictors, a tree-based algorithm is first built as previously described for the age–BMI problem except that now each partitioning step considers all possible splits of the data by all potential predictors. Suppose the dataset contains p predictors denoted $X_1, \ldots, X_p$ and a continuous outcome Y. For each predictor X_i, the algorithm splits the observations into two groups $X_i \leq c$ and $X_i > c$ for some cutoff c and calculates a value $\Delta(i, c)$ that indicates how well this partition (of the ith predictor using cutoff c) improves the predictive performance. Most often, as in our example, $\Delta(i, c)$ is defined as the reduction in MSE corresponding to partitioning the data by splitting X_i at c. Each split is chosen to yield the partition that maximizes $\Delta(i, c)$. The tree is grown and pruned in accordance with the tuning parameters, which are selected by cross-validation.

As an example, we predict total annual medical expenditures in the MEPS 2017 data given the predictors in Table 10.1 plus total expenditures in 2016. Figure 10.11 shows the cross-validation results of fitting trees of various sizes that would result from different specifications for the pruning parameter α. The x-axis shows the size of the tree, and the y-axis shows the relative performance (i.e., the MSE relative to the trivial tree with one node containing all observations) estimated by 10-fold cross-validation. The mean relative performance and one standard error around it are presented for each tree size. We see that there is a sharp initial improvement in performance and then a plateau, which is followed by a steady increase in the relative MSE, with larger trees performing no better than the optimal tree with eight nodes.

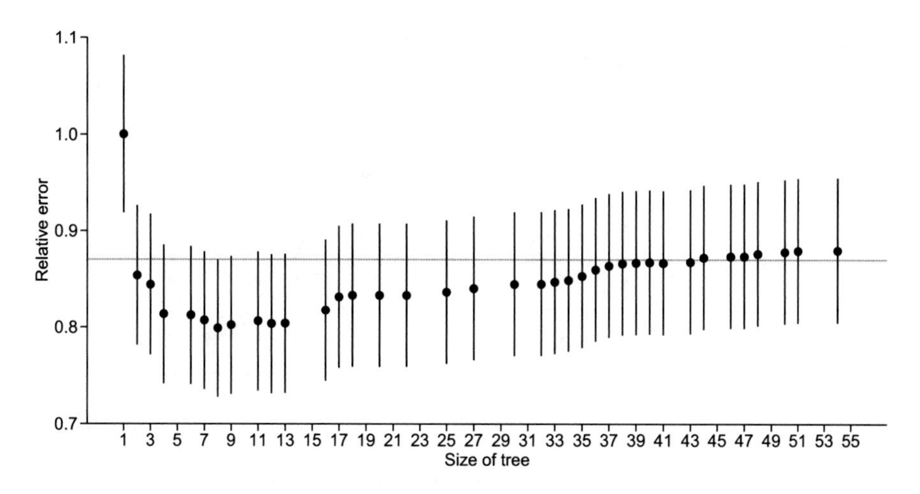

Fig. 10.11 Predictive performance for trees of different sizes for total expenditures in 2017 from the MEPS 2016–2017 panel data. The orange horizontal line indicates the smallest value of the relative error plus one standard error

Figure 10.12 shows the fitted regression tree with eight terminal nodes. The most important variable for prediction is total expenditures in 2016; it is the variable used for the first three splits. After that, the splits are by perceived health status, insurance coverage, total expenditures in 2016 again, and finally age. Note that these latter splits are not across all observations; they are only for the subjects in the parent nodes. For example, the partition by type of insurance coverage is only for the 2% of the observations whose total expenditures in 2016 were greater than $40,221. Similarly, the partition by perceived health status is only for the subset of individuals whose total expenditures in 2016 were in the range of $11,005–$40,221, amounting to 9% of the total sample. Although 26 predictors were considered, the regression tree uses only 4 for prediction. The tree groups observations according to the combinations of predictor values corresponding to each terminal node, and the predictions are simply given by the average outcome in each group. Thus, the tree in Fig. 10.12 only produces eight distinct predicted values, and these are summarized in Table 10.2.

10.6.3 Classification Trees

When the outcome is binary or categorical, having two or more classes, the aim of prediction is to classify each observation into its correct class based on the predictors. In classification problems, the predictive accuracy is not measured by the MSE because, in general, classes do not have a numerical interpretation. Instead, a different measure of performance more suited to classification problems is used. A

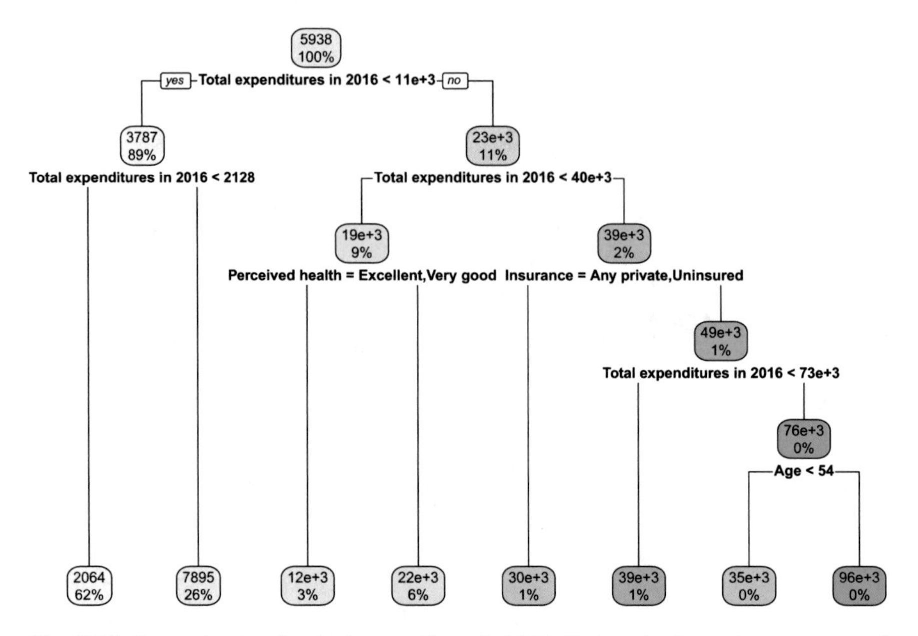

Fig. 10.12 Regression tree for total expenditures in 2017. Each node shows the percentage of observations from the sample included in it and their predicted expenditures in 2017, calculated by the average expenditure among observations at that node

Table 10.2 Predictions from regression tree for total medical expenditures in 2017 for persons age 18 years or older given variables observed in MEPS 2016 data

Costs in 2016	Perceived health	Insurance	Age	Predicted in 2017
\$0–\$2127	Any	Any	Any	\$2064
\$2128–\$11,004	Any	Any	Any	\$7895
\$11,005–\$40,221	Excellent, very good	Any	Any	\$12,186
\$11,005–\$40,221	Good, fair, poor	Any	Any	\$22,149
>\$40,221	Any	Any private, uninsured	Any	\$29,884
\$40,222–\$72,906	Any	Public only	Any	\$39,288
>\$72,906	Any	Public only	18–53	\$35,261
>\$72,906	Any	Public only	54–85	\$95,723

natural measure is the *misclassification error*, that is, the number of observations classified incorrectly.

Any predictive algorithm, including regression trees, can be used for classification. A classification tree is grown and pruned in the same way, and with the same tuning parameters as a regression tree. The prediction is again calculated over the terminal nodes of the tree; the predicted value for any given node is the majority class among observations at that node.

Figure 10.13 shows the classification tree for the event of any hospitalization in 2017 based on the predictors in Table 10.1. The root node at the top tells us

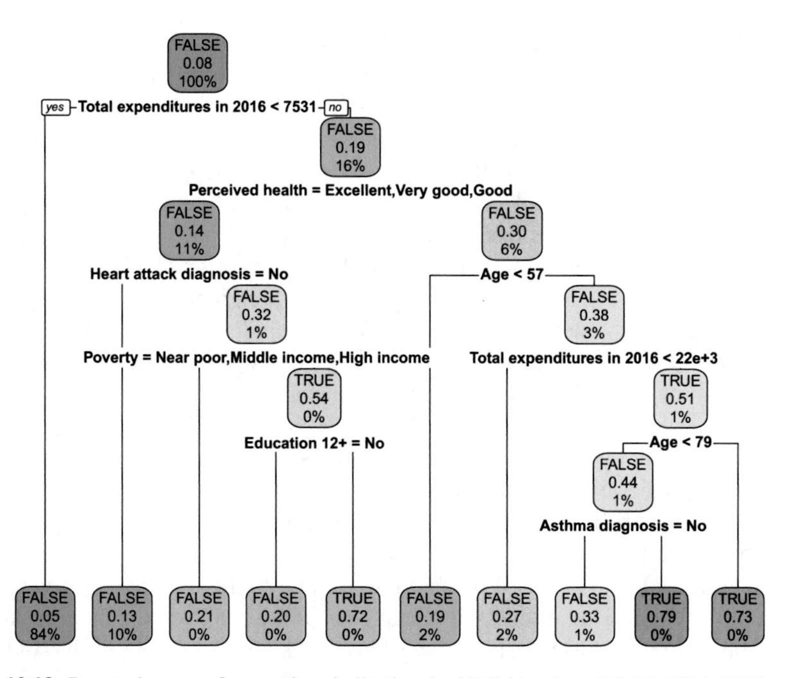

Fig. 10.13 Regression tree for any hospitalization in 2017 based on MEPS 2016–2017 panel data. Each terminal node shows the prediction (TRUE for hospitalization and FALSE for no hospitalization), proportions of individuals in that subset who were hospitalized in 2017, and the percentage of individuals in the subset

that only 8% (actually 7.6%) of individuals were hospitalized in 2017. As for the prediction of total expenditures in 2017, the first split is by total expenditures in 2016; those spending less than $7531 in 2016 (84% of the sample) are predicted not to be hospitalized in 2017. (In fact, only 5% of these subjects were hospitalized in 2017.) The remainder of the sample (16%) were variously subdivided based on perceived health, prior diagnosis of heart attack, family income, year of education, age, and prior diagnosis of asthma. In the end, the algorithm predicted that three subsets of individuals will be hospitalized in 2017: (1) those with total expenditures in 2016 at least $7531 perceived to have at least good health, prior diagnosis of heart attack, low income or poor, and 12 or more years of education; (2) those age 57–79 years with total expenditures in 2016 of at least $21,558 perceived to have fair or poor health and prior diagnosis with asthma; and (3) those age 79–85 years with total expenditures in 2016 of at least $21,558 perceived to have fair or poor health.

Classification algorithms do not directly classify observations. Instead, they predict the probability of the outcome being in each possible class. Our regularization example predicting hospitalization was actually a classification problem in which the predicted outcome was the probability of hospitalization in 2017. To produce a binary prediction from a predicted probability requires thresholding that probability. For binary trees, the probability is presented for the positive outcome (here, being hospitalized in 2017) and thresholded at 0.5. Thus, when the predicted probability is larger than 0.5, the algorithm predicts class "TRUE" (hospitalization), and when it is smaller than 0.5, it predicts class "FALSE."

Based on this threshold, the misclassification error of the tree in Fig. 10.13 is 7.2%. But naive classification of all individuals as not hospitalized has a misclassification error of only 7.6%! It is often difficult to classify rare events, as the majority of the observations are in one of the classes, and simply predicting all individuals as being in the larger class can yield apparently reasonable performance.

There are at least two ways to deal with classification problems with rare events. First, a larger tree can be grown in the hope of finding small groups in which hospitalization is more frequent. However, this increases the complexity of the tree and the risk of overfitting. Second, different weights can be assigned to different types of misclassification errors. For example, predicting that a person will be hospitalized in the next year when he/she will not (a false positive) may be less costly than predicting a person will not be hospitalized when he/she will (a false negative). Giving different weights to different misclassification errors can change both the construction of the tree and the final prediction. This second approach should be considered on a case-by-case basis, and it is appropriate only when there is indeed a difference between the implications of false positives and false negatives. When predicting health care utilization and costs, the two types of misclassification errors often have different implications, so direct examination of these individual error rates may be more relevant for evaluating prediction accuracy than the overall misclassification error rate even when event of interest is not rare.

10.7 Ensemble Methods: Random Forests

Classification and regression trees produce results with large variance. If two trees are constructed from two independent samples taken from the same population, a large difference between the results is expected due to differences in splits close to the root node. Single trees are rarely competitive in terms of predictive performance; however ensembles of trees, as described in this chapter, are powerful predictive methods.

To address the variance issue, one remedy would be to draw many independent samples, estimate a tree for each, and average the results. Specifically, for a new individual, predict their outcome within each tree, and average these results to produce the final prediction. This will reduce the variance of the predicted outcome, but it is not practical. Instead, we can apply the idea of bootstrapping discussed in Chap. 7. Specifically, we can generate many bootstrap samples from the data and grow a tree for each. While the samples are not independent, they are different enough to gain considerable reduction in variance. This approach is referred to as *bagging* (bootstrapping and aggregating). One disadvantage of bagging is that moderately important predictors may not be detected because more important predictors, identified early, may dominate across the bootstrapped samples. This makes the trees constructed by bagging too similar to one another.

To enhance independence of the trees grown using bootstrap samples, we can go a step further. At each split, rather than considering all p predictors, we consider only a random collection of $m < p$ predictors. By randomly selecting different predictors for each split, variables other than the most important ones have an opportunity to be entered into the final prediction. The enhanced algorithm that combines bagging with random predictor selection at each split is appropriately called a *random forest* [7]. In a random forest, averaging across trees helps to address our usual concerns about the overfitting of a single tree. In addition, growing larger trees enables more predictors to be involved in the splitting, permitting deeper investigation of the data. Therefore, in random forest algorithms, the trees are grown to be quite large, often until all individuals in each terminal node have the same values for all of their predictors.

In a dataset with n observations and p potential predictors, the random forest algorithm consists of the following steps:

1. Generate B (say $B = 500$) bootstrap samples from the data. A bootstrap sample is drawn by sampling with replacement n new observations from the data. Sampling with replacement means that several observations will be present more than once in the sample and others will be completely absent.
2. For each sample, construct a regression or classification tree as appropriate. However, instead of considering all predictors at each split, randomly sample m from the p potential predictors, and grow the tree starting with the best possible split among the m selected predictors. A common practice is to take $m = \sqrt{p}$ for classification problems and $m = p/3$ for regression problems. For example, for $p = 25$, each split uses $m = 5$ random predictors if the task is classification.
3. Combine the predictions from the resulting B trees into a single value by using the average prediction across the trees.

Random forests can be fit in R using the package `randomForest` [8]. We compare the performance of a random forest predictor to that of a single tree in the regression and classification problems analyzed earlier in this chapter using the MEPS data. We randomly split the data into training and test datasets comprising 70% and 30% of the observations, respectively. We then fit both algorithms to the training data—this involves first identifying the best tuning/flexibility parameters by cross-validation—and then comparing the predictive performance using the test data. For the continuous outcome (total expenditures in 2017), the performance in the test data is measured using the MSE, i.e., the mean squared difference between the predicted and actual expenditures in 2017. For the binary outcome (hospitalization in 2017), the performance in the test data is measured using the misclassification error rate.

For either outcome, we grow random forests of 500 trees. There is no simple way to present the trees and their predictions. To evaluate the performance of the algorithm, each observation in the test data is predicted by averaging the predictions from each of the 500 trees. For predicting total expenditures in 2017, the random forest MSE is 151999462 compared to 161732697 for a single regression tree, a 6% improvement.

Applying a random forest to predict hospitalization in 2017 results in 8.1% misclassification error rate in the test data, which is similar to the 8.2% misclassification error rate of a single tree. Both results are poor, however, since 7.6% of individuals were hospitalized in 2017, so a naive classifier that predicts no individuals are hospitalized performs better than either. Predicting a rare event is challenging; see Chen et al. [9] for two modifications of random forests when the outcome is extremely unbalanced.

While a random forest is a true black-box algorithm, there have been attempts to extract the importance of the predictors used by the algorithm. There are different ways to quantify importance, but they all relate to how the predictor improves accuracy. One commonly used approach quantifies how each predictor contributes to the performance of each tree using the observations not selected by the bootstrap sample—known as *out-of-bag* (OOB) observations. To quantify the importance of a predictor X, the performance of each tree in the random forest is measured twice in predicting the outcomes for the corresponding OOB sample. First, the accuracy of the fitted tree is measured in the OOB sample. Second, the accuracy is measured again after randomly shuffling the predictor X across the OOB observations. The importance of X is calculated by measuring the difference in accuracy; if X is not important, the two accuracy measurements will be similar. The importance measures for each predictor are averaged over the trees, and a graphical display can be generated to visualize their rankings.

Figure 10.14 presents this measure of importance for the predictors in the random forest for total expenditures in 2017. Total expenditures in 2016 are the most important predictor, followed by age and prior diagnosis of high blood pressure. However, this measure of importance should be interpreted with caution when

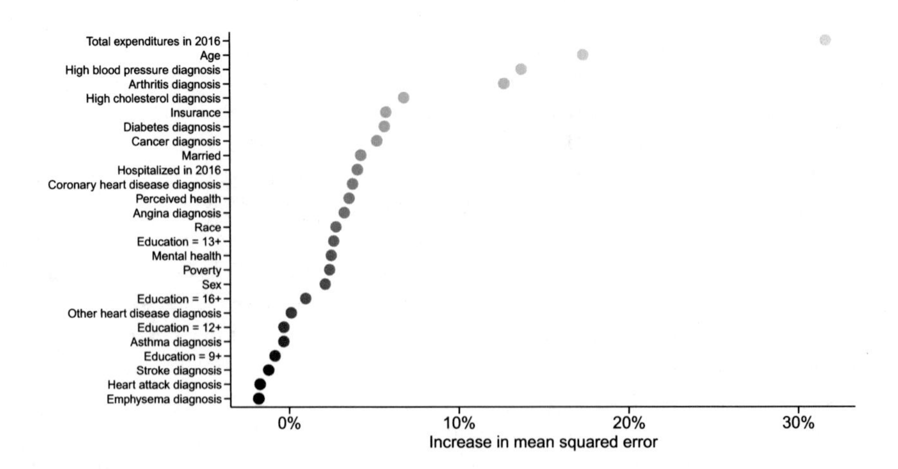

Fig. 10.14 Importance of predictors in a random forest to predict total expenditures in 2017 using longitudinal MEPS 2016–2017 panel data

it comes to hypotheses or questions about specific predictors and their role in explaining variation in the outcome. If one wants to understand the effect of covariates on the outcome and not purely predict its values, it may be appropriate to move from the algorithms culture to the models culture and harness the methods from previous chapters.

A random forest is an example of an ensemble learning method. Ensemble learning methods combine the predictions from multiple algorithms. In the case of random forests, all the component prediction algorithms are the same—either classification or regression trees. However, there is no reason why this should be the case. Indeed, the idea of averaging predictions across several models applies regardless of the type of model. *Ensemble learning* is a term used to describe this general idea. Ensemble methods fit many prediction models to the same data and combine them, harnessing the wisdom of the crowd of techniques to determine the predicted value. Each component model has strengths and weaknesses in its ability to accurately predict the outcome. The hope is that when we combine the models, the strengths will yield a final prediction that is more accurate than any single component. Many learning techniques are based on this idea; they differ mainly in the ways they fit and combine the models.

10.8 Summary

We titled this chapter "Prediction" to emphasize its focus on predictive algorithms. The predictive algorithms and analytics discussed in this chapter represent only a small part of the larger field of data science. The field of data science is multidisciplinary with considerable overlap with computer science and machine learning.

Breiman's paper on two cultures was a powerful and timely exhortation to the statistical community to broaden its perspective and embrace the algorithms culture. The big data revolution has turned this into an imperative, particularly in the "large p" setting. With prediction problems based on thousands and even millions of pieces of information, automated algorithms are essential. The field of statistical learning brings machine learning and statistics together. Yet, even as the statistical field has adapted and integrated algorithmic methods, it has not abandoned traditional inferential goals and principles; witness the growing areas of post-selection inference and targeted learning [10–13], which address inference based on data-adaptive models and aim to make inferences about the data-generating mechanism.

Classical regression models are restricted to a very specific formulation of the associations between the predictors and the outcome (generally, linear and additive or multiplicative relationships). Of course, this is not guaranteed to hold, even approximately. Predictive methods are generally freed from this constraint, assuming only that there is some functional relationship with only minimal restrictions. A prediction method performs well if it can recover the link between the predictors and the outcome no matter the underlying form of the association. However, this task can only be achieved in general if the sample size is sufficiently large.

Despite the power of predictive methods, there are important caveats. First, not all problems require the machinery of predictive algorithms. If the dataset is small, comprised of tens or hundreds of observations with relatively few covariates, it may be preferable to restrict the model using subject-matter knowledge instead of fitting a flexible black-box algorithm. We do not recommend letting any algorithm run blindly—be sure that relevant predictors are used, that categorical variables are coded correctly, that missing data are addressed, and that the algorithm used is suitable for the outcome. It is critical to understand the tuning parameters and recognize the limitations of a predictive model.

When the Heritage Health Prize was announced, the organizers envisioned the final predictive model being harnessed to generate "new care plans and strategies to reach patients before emergencies occur, thereby reducing the number of unnecessary hospitalizations." In fact, this is a goal of explaining rather than predicting. To prevent unnecessary hospitalizations, it is not enough to know who is at high risk; we also need to know why.

10.9 Software and Data

R code to download data and to carry out the examples in this book is available at the GitHub page https://roman-gulati.github.io/statistics-for-health-data-science/. In addition to the R packages cited in Chap. 1, this chapter also used the `RColorBrewer` [14], `randomForest` [8], `glmnet` [15], `rattle` [16], `rpart` [17], and `rpart.plot` [18] packages.

References

1. Flom, P.: (2018). https://medium.com/@peterflom
2. Breiman, L.: Statistical modeling: the two cultures (with comments and a rejoinder by the author). Stat. Sci. **16**(3), 199–231 (2001a)
3. for Disease Control, C.: Prevention: national health and nutrition examination survey. https://www.cdc.gov/nchs/nhanes/index.htm. Accessed 12 February 2020
4. James, G., Witten, D., Hastie, T., Tibshirani, R.: An Introduction to Statistical Learning with Applications in R. Springer, Berlin (2013). https://faculty.marshall.usc.edu/gareth-james/ISL/
5. for Healthcare Research, A.: Quality: Medical Expenditure Panel Survey (). http://www.ahrq.gov/research/data/meps/index.html. Accessed 12 February 2020
6. Breiman, L., Friedman, J.H., Olshen, R.A., Stone, C.J.: Classification and Regression Trees. Wadsworth and Brooks, Mason (1984)
7. Breiman, L.: Random forests. Mach. Learn. **45**(1), 5–32 (2001b)
8. Liaw, A., Wiener, M.: Classification and regression by randomForest. R News **2**(3), 18–22 (2002). https://CRAN.R-project.org/doc/Rnews/

9. Chen, C., Liaw, A., Breiman, L.: Using random forest to learn imbalanced data. Tech. Rep. 666, University of California, Berkeley (2004). https://statistics.berkeley.edu/tech-reports/666
10. van der Laan, M.J., Rose, S.: Targeted Learning: Causal Inference for Observational and Experimental Data. Springer, Berlin (2011)
11. Lee, J., Sun, D., Sun, Y., Taylor, J.: Exact post-selection inference with application to the lasso. Ann. Stat. **44**, 907–927 (2016)
12. Tibshirani, R.J., Taylor, J., Lockhart, R., Tibshirani, R.: Exact post-selection inference for sequential regression procedures. J. Am. Stat. Assoc. **111**, 600–620 (2016)
13. Hyun, S., G'sell, M., Tibshirani, R.: Exact post-selection inference for the generalized lasso path. Electron. J. Stat. **12**, 1053–1097 (2018)
14. Neuwirth, E.: RColorBrewer: ColorBrewer palettes (2014). https://CRAN.R-project.org/package=RColorBrewer. R package version 1.1-2
15. Friedman, J., Hastie, T., Tibshirani, R.: Regularization paths for generalized linear models via coordinate descent. J. Stat. Softw. **33**(1), 1–22 (2010). http://www.jstatsoft.org/v33/i01/
16. Williams, G.J.: Data Mining with Rattle and R: The Art of Excavating Data for Knowledge Discovery. Springer, Berlin (2011)
17. Therneau, T., Atkinson, B.: rpart: Recursive partitioning and regression trees (2019). https://CRAN.R-project.org/package=rpart. R package version 4.1-15
18. Milborrow, S.: rpart.plot: Plot 'rpart' Models: an enhanced version of 'plot.rpart' (2019). https://CRAN.R-project.org/package=rpart.plot. R package version 3.0.8

Index

R. Etzioni et al., *Statistics for Health Data Science*, Springer Texts in Statistics,
https://doi.org/10.1007/978-3-030-59889-1